HEALTH IS WEALTH

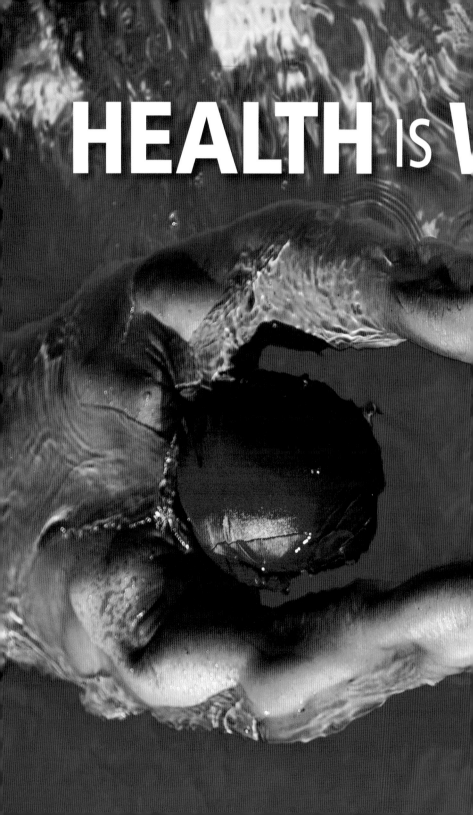

EALTH

ERFORMANCE NUTRITION
FOR THE COMPETITIVE EDGE

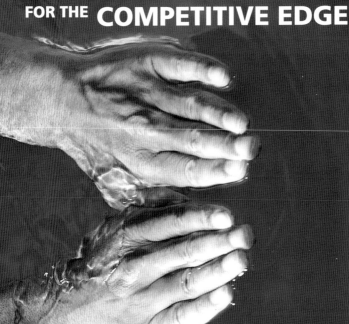

By
Louis Ignarro, Ph.D.
(1998 Nobel Laureate in Medicine
and author of *NO More Heart Disease)*

and

Andrew Myers, N.D.
(author of *Simple Health Value*)

Health Is Wealth
Performance Nutrition for the Competitive Edge

by Louis Ignarro, Ph.D. and Andrew Myers, N.D.

Published by Health Value Publications

Cover Design by Cari Campbell, Cari Campbell Design
Interior Design by Nick Zelinger, NZ Graphics

International Standard Book Number 13: 978-1-61389-002-8

Warning-Disclaimer

Health Value Publications and Drs. Ignarro and Myers have designed this book to provide information in regard to the subject matter covered. It is sold with the understanding that the publisher and author are not liable for the misconception or misuse of information provided. Every effort has been made to make this book as complete and accurate as possible. The purpose of this book is to educate. The authors and Health Value Publications shall have neither liability nor responsibility to any person or entity with respect to loss, damage, or injury caused or alleged to be caused directly or indirectly by the information contained in this book. The information presented herein is in no way intended as a substitute for medical counseling.

It is recommended that you do not self-diagnose. Proper medical care is critical to good health. If you have symptoms suggestive of an illness, please consult a physician—preferably a naturopath, holistic physician, osteopath, chiropractor, or other natural health care specialist. If you are currently taking a prescription medication, you absolutely must consult your doctor before discontinuing it.

The Nobel Prize is a registered trademark of The Nobel Foundation. The image pictured on the cover of Health Is Wealth is Dr. Ignarro's actual prize awarded to him in 1998.

The Nobel Foundation has no affiliation with the authors in regards to this book and has not reviewed, approved, or endorsed the content of Health Is Wealth.

For more information, visit healthiswealth.net.

We dedicate this book to all athletes
who aspire to perform at their personal best
and to our families and friends for their love and support.

Contents

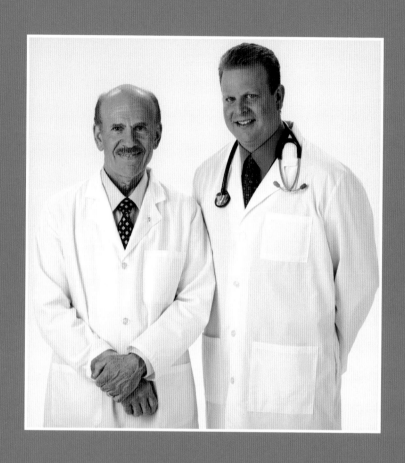

Introduction

YOU'RE AN ATHLETE. YOU TRAIN HARD. You try to eat a balanced diet—rich in lean protein, healthy fats, whole grains, fruits, and vegetables—in order to be healthy and fuel muscle growth and endurance. You follow the latest in training science so you can slice a few seconds off your 10K time, lift a few more pounds on the bench press, or gain those last few inches in your vertical leap that will let you finally—*finally*—dunk a basketball. Whether you're a weekend warrior, collegiate athlete, or professional, your goal is the same: wring peak performance from your body again and again, while avoiding injury.

But how do you make it happen? How do the world's elite athletes make their bodies put out such incredible speed, power, or endurance? What do they know that you don't? Is there a secret?

Yes. The truth is that optimal athletic performance isn't just about natural talent or relentless training. It's about *nutrition*. Specifically, it's about supplementing your diet with the right nutrients to fuel your performance. We call them Power Nutrients. While you may believe you can get all the nutrients you need to perform at your best from the food you eat, the truth is that it's nearly impossible to do so. Even if your diet is nearly perfect, you may still be missing some of the key nutrients that science has shown are critical to supercharging your speed, strength, explosiveness, coordination, and endurance.

That's why we wrote this book. In its pages are the secrets of ten Power Nutrients that will unlock your athletic potential. You'll learn how these nutrients work at the cellular level to make your muscles, nerves, bones, heart, and cardiovascular system—every part of your body—function more efficiently. Want to reach the next level? Want to set a new personal best in your next triathlon or keep from "bonking"—hitting the wall—on your next 60-mile ride? We've got the answers.

Why Supplementation Matters

If you aren't supplementing your diet every day, with nutrients that fuel your body's well-being at the cellular level, then you are leaving performance on the table. It's that simple. Of course, if you don't know this, you're not alone. Our own research and numerous outside studies indicate that many top athletes—even professional athletes—aren't aware of the importance of proper supplementation. They admit they don't understand what the proper nutritional supplements are for them. So, don't feel too bad if your supplementation up until now has consisted of a daily multivitamin—or nothing at all.

Here's the big picture: whole-body health and optimal performance of all the body's systems can only be achieved when the cells are functioning at their peak. As a huge body of emerging research is revealing, this is most likely to occur when cellular nutrition is optimized and nitric oxide (NO) is abundant in the body. NO is the heart and soul of this book. It is the nutrient that underlies the superlative performance of virtually every major system in the body.

Together with exercise and a healthy diet, supplementation boosts your cellular levels of NO, leading to increased circulation, improved oxygenation, and more efficient fueling of tissues, and, in the end, improved energy and athletic output. Combined, they form the Peak Performance Loop, which looks like this:

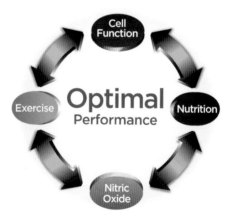

This loop is the core of peak athletic performance. When you provide your body with the proper array of nutrients, it produces more NO and utilizes it with greater effectiveness, which vastly enhances the condition of the cells that form each body system. Because of this, your cells are able to function closer to their optimal levels. Meanwhile, exercise increases NO levels, and the cycle continues. The end result: peak athletic performance and greater foundational wellness.

What do we mean by cellular function related to exercise? Muscle cells make muscle fibers contract faster and longer to deliver strength, explosiveness (e.g., jumping in basketball), speed, and power. Nerve cells conduct electrical impulses to the muscles and joints, providing for quick reflexes and fast reaction time. Osteocytes, or bone cells, provide the foundation for muscle attachment and give the body strength and solidity. The cells of the digestive system break down food and absorb nutrients. Red blood cells carry oxygen and fuel to the muscles and organs. Lymph cells clear waste products. Individual cells, working in concert, produce everything your body does. When cell function is at its peak, so is performance.

Think of the diagram as a table, viewed from the top. Take away one ingredient—one leg—and the whole thing topples. Supplementation with Power Nutrients works in tandem with exercise and proper diet to maximize your NO levels and give you everything your body needs to respond to the demands you're placing on it.

The 3D Effect

Without supplementation…well, you may already know what happens. Are you frustrated that more training doesn't lead to better performance? Are you feeling sluggish or mentally cloudy? Do you find yourself getting injured more often than you should? There's a reason: you're not giving your body the nutrients it needs. Because you're an athlete, you need more robust nutrition than the average "couch potato." You ask a lot of your body on training days, game days, or race days. Your diet just isn't getting the job done. Without proper supplementation to provide cellular nutrition, many athletes find themselves suffering from what we call the **3D Effect**.

We introduced this nutritional concept in our first book, *Health Is Wealth* (www.healthiswealth.net). It describes the three stages of **Nutrient Deficiency Syndrome**, a process that occurs when the body falls short of sufficient levels of certain crucial nutrients. The 3D Effect consists of the following progressive stages:

1. **Depletion**—Each biological system requires minimal levels of certain nutrients to function properly. When you don't take in

enough of a specific nutrient, the systems that depend on that nutrient will cannibalize other systems to get enough of it to continue operating—in essence, robbing Peter to pay Paul. Eventually, without replenishment, those nutrient stores will run dry. When that happens, you cross into deficiency.

2. **Deficiency**—This occurs when the chronic depletion of one or more essential nutrients begin to cause the breakdown of one or more body systems at the cellular level. You may not experience any symptoms of this breakdown yet, but it's still occurring. Unchecked, this leads to dysfunction.

3. **Dysfunction**—At this stage, enough cellular damage has accumulated that you begin to experience symptoms of what doctors call "disease." People with dysfunction in their muscular systems may experience muscle pain, while people with cardiac dysfunction may feel chest pain or shortness of breath, for example. Because symptoms seem to have appeared overnight, this is the stage that conventional wisdom regards as the beginning of disease, but, in reality, it is the endpoint of a multistage process that can last for years and begins with a simple lack of proper nutrients.

For an athlete, there is a fourth type of "D"—**Diminished Performance**. Rather than experiencing the symptoms of heart disease or arthritis, you notice that you can't seem to perform at the level you want. You can't increase your speed or endurance. You can't jump as high or lift as much weight as you once could. You seem to get injured easier and recover slower. Your body hits the wall.

The good news about the 3D Effect is that it can be reversed—and the reversal is a simple matter. Just re-introduce sufficient supplies of needed key Power Nutrients into your body through supplementation (based on your unique biochemical profile and the demands of your sport and your lifestyle, of course); and you will see your symptoms resolve and your body begin to feel and perform at the level at which it's capable. *Health is Wealth: Performance Nutrition* is all about showing you exactly how to do that.

Who This Book Is For

In the second section of this book, you're going to read candid interviews with some of the most finely-tuned athletes the world has to offer: ultra-endurance runners, Ironman™ champions, English channel swimmers, mountaineers, and so on. But that doesn't mean that *Health Is Wealth: Performance Nutrition* is only for the elite professional or Olympic-caliber athlete. It is far from it.

We created this book to educate any active, athletic individual—from the ambitious weekend athlete to the dedicated gym rat to the serious age-group triathlete—in the ways that proper nutrition from supplementation can optimize athletic performance, improve recovery and resistance to injury, and enhance overall health and wellness in the long term. The group of readers for whom this book is ideal and what they will get from it is described below:

- For **weekend warriors** who play everything from softball to soccer to tennis at an intense level, *Health Is Wealth: Performance Nutrition* is your key to foods and supplements that will help you do more, outplay the other guy, and avoid the nagging pulls and strains that come with age.

- For **dedicated exercisers** who workout 5-6 days per week and pride themselves on their fitness and health, *Health Is Wealth: Performance Nutrition* offers information on improving lifelong health as you age, while making you resistant to injuries and boosting your results in the gym.

- For **weight lifters** who spend hours at the gym, *Health Is Wealth: Performance Nutrition* brings insights about NO, as well as other supplements that can enhance your ability to build muscle, shed fat, and become stronger…longer.

- For **serious amateur athletes** who race bikes, run marathons, compete in Ironman™, or perform any other physical activity that takes up many hours each week, *Health Is Wealth: Performance Nutrition* provides invaluable, scientific research into foods and critical micronutrients that can optimize your recovery, increase your muscular endurance, improve explosiveness and speed, and keep you going when other competitors stop.

- For **professional- and international-caliber athletes (and those who aspire to be)**, *Health Is Wealth: Performance Nutrition* is a hard-science guide to nutrients that most other elite athletes are not using—100% legal substances that can give you an edge by making sure your body is operating at its peak and repairing the damage you inflict upon it through the demands of your sport.

In short, this book can help athletes of any level, from Olympians and pros to the ambitious amateur who wants to be better, get more out of his or her body, and excel in his or her chosen sport, while doing more to stay healthy and active longer.

Why Aren't Athletes Doing This?

It's shocking just how many athletes overlook this critical component to optimal performance, which is something they can easily add into their daily routine. We interviewed world-class professional and amateur athletes, from Ironman™ champions to Major League Baseball Hall of Famers, and they told us time and time again that not only did they not take much in the way of nutritional supplements, but they didn't know what NO was or what it did. One marathoner told us that her nutrition plan was based on the food pyramid she learned in third grade!

This is part of an alarming trend. A survey of Finnish athletes, published in the *Journal of the International Society of Sports Nutrition*, suggests that supplement use among Olympic athletes has been dropping. According to the survey, in 2002, 81% of surveyed athletes used dietary supplements; in

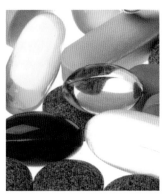

2009, only 73% did—an 8% reduction. The report suggests that purity concerns, as well as worries about overconsumption of certain nutrients, might lie behind the decline.

In an article in the *New York Times* from early 2010, athletes were asked about supplementation. While many said they understood the need for nutrients, they were hesitant to add pills or powders to their daily routine. Female athletes were open to multivitamins, energy drinks, and nutrient bars, but were reluctant to take supplements.

Some of this hesitation comes from not understanding exactly which supplements are best—which boost performance and energy versus those that create "expensive pee," as critics of supplementation like to call it. In our opinion, that's self-defeating ignorance.

Science shows that proper nutrition at the cellular level is at least as important to both health and athletic performance as strength training, cardiovascular training, and recovery time. In fact, it's the foundation for everything else. When you've trained as hard as you can, supplementing your diet with Power Nutrients designed specifically to boost muscle growth, recovery, circulation, energy efficiency, and resilience of muscle fibers and connective tissue makes all the difference.

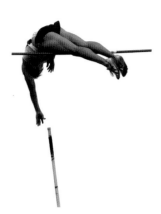

Nitric Oxide: Just Short of Miraculous

The ten Power Nutrients we will discuss in detail later in this book have a common thread: they affect your body's ability to make or use NO more effectively. This is no small matter. NO is a gaseous signaling molecule—not to be confused with nitrous oxide, also called "laughing gas," which we recommend you avoid unless you're at the dentist's—that, when released into your body, causes your blood vessels to dilate, allowing more blood, oxygen, and nutrients to reach even the most remote tissues. It's not hard to see how this would positively impact athletic performance and also promote cardiovascular health. In fact, the pioneering research into NO's incredible impact on cardiovascular health earned Dr. Louis Ignarro, the coauthor of this book, the Nobel Prize in Medicine in 1998.

Further research has shown that NO is useful for more than optimal cardiovascular performance and healthy coronary arteries. Now, it appears that this molecule has beneficial effects on nearly every tissue in your body, allowing them to combat disease more effectively, improve performance and endurance, and enhance overall health. NO is one of the most important substances in the human body: it is the closest thing to a miracle for promoting wellness and athletic excellence that science has ever found. Yet, you may never have heard about it.

In his ongoing research since winning the Nobel Prize, Dr. Ignarro has found that, with all the myriad benefits of regular exercise, the greatest benefit for over-all health may be that exercise dramatically increases the body's sustained levels of NO. When you perform a routine of intensive exercise and then add a regimen of Power Nutrients that either boost NO production, increase NO's effectiveness, or protect NO from being broken down chemically, you have an enormously powerful prescription for enhancing athletic performance, preventing disease, and promoting general wellness. It's also a prescription that is low-cost, virtually free of negative side effects, and extremely effective for people at all levels of athletic activity.

NO is the wonder molecule that ties together the benefits of exercise, diet, and supplementation. Increasing and maintaining high levels of NO in your body will give you what you need to reach your next level of athletic perform-ance—and we're going to explain to you how to get there by supplementing your diet with ten critical Power Nutrients. By reading this material, you'll increase your **NO IQ** and learn the nutritional secrets to peak performance that even some world-class pro athletes don't know.

Study Links Nitric Oxide and Stamina

Research conducted at the University of Exeter revealed that taking dietary supplements to boost NO in the body significantly boosts stamina during high-intensity exercise. When athletes con-sumed a dietary supplement of beetroot juice, which has a high nitrate content that boosts NO, their bodies began using oxygen more efficiently during exercise, leading to a striking increase in performance. The study indicated that endurance athletes could exer-cise up to 20% longer and produce a 1-2% improvement in race times.

Source: Nutrition Industry Executive, October 2010

A Growing Body of Solid Research

Our work is active and ongoing. We continue to review new research on nutrient interactions within the body's biochemical pathways and physiological systems. Our studies have uncovered the vital relationships between specific nutrients—protein, amino acids, antioxidants, and many more—and healthy tissues. Their relationships demonstrate an unmistakable link between nutrient supplementation, NO levels, and optimal performance. We're also athletes ourselves, so we have first-hand insight into the types of practical, in-game "returns on investment" that athletes are seeking.

The result is a simple, back-to-basics approach that's also a revolution. So, whether you read this while you're on your trainer, putting in your time on the elliptical machine at the gym, or taking a break from a lifting or stretching session, spend a few hours and raise your **Performance Nutrition IQ**. It could be the best thing you ever do for your body, health, and athletic performance.

Dr. Louis Ignarro
Dr. Andrew Myers

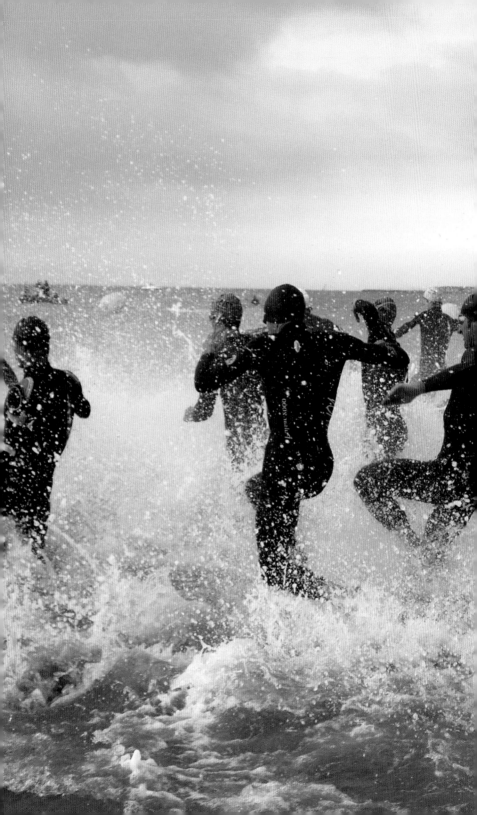

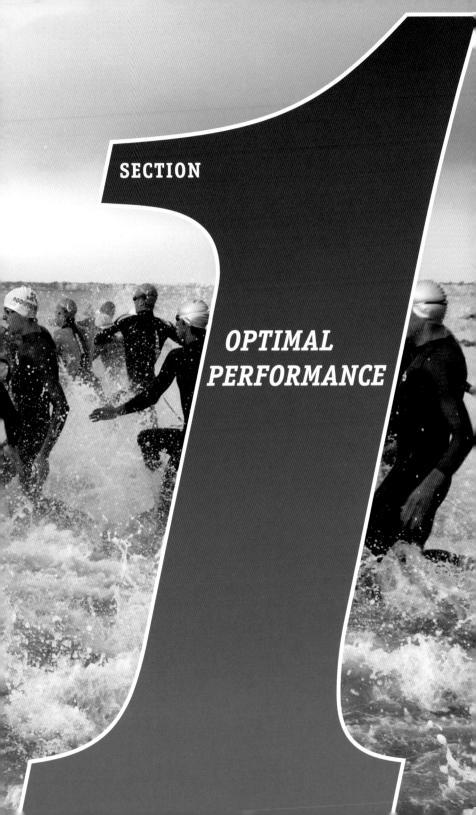

SECTION

1

OPTIMAL
PERFORMANCE

Chapter One
Trillions of Incredible Machines

"As I see it, every day you do one of two things: build health or produce disease in yourself."
—*Adelle Davis, Nutritionist*

If properly cared for, and nourished by the full range of vital nutrients, the human body has the ability to live with health and vitality for 100 years, perhaps more. Unfortunately, many of us don't give our bodies the nutrients they require. Even athletes, who believe they are keenly attuned to their bodies' needs, fall short here. You may believe that supplementing a healthy and varied diet with nutrition bars and electrolyte drinks is enough to ensure peak performance. Unfortunately, this is not the case.

Getting the most out of your body requires taking a whole-body view of nutrition, not just "sports nutrition." Sports nutrition is a somewhat nebulous term, which is more about marketing than science. We prefer the concept of performance nutrition, which includes enriching every part of your body with the full range of vital nutrients.

Whole-body nutrition is a philosophy that focuses on restoring and maintaining the complete function of each and every one of the trillions of cells in your body over your entire lifetime. How well your cells operate determines how your muscles, bones, organs, and other systems perform when you place demands on them, and these control whether you get the athletic performance you aspire to or fall short. So, let's look at a cell and see why it craves the nutrients it does.

The Complex Dance of Your Cells

The average adult human body contains trillions of cells. The body of an average 70 kilogram (165 lb.) healthy male at 50 years of age is composed of:

- 60 trillion cells
- 15 trillion red blood cells (25% of all cells)
- 6 trillion *vascular endothelial* cells (10% of all cells).

Each of those cells are basically a microscopic power plant that uses mitochondria to convert food energy into chemical energy. Depending on the cell's structure and its role in the body, it will use that energy for specific purposes—the electrical energy that carries the messages over the neural connections in your brain, the chemical energy that contracts your muscle fibers so you can shoot a basketball or pedal a bike, and so on.

Exercise at any level—from walking to the mailbox to running a marathon—requires cells to work together in perfect coordination and involves virtually every system of the body. This is a gross over-simplification of the biochemical processes that take place, but think about returning a serve in tennis. First, your eyes have to focus on the tennis ball traveling toward you and relay the reflected light to your brain, where your visual cortex translates that information into, "She just hit a serve to your backhand." Then, your brain sends signals through your central nervous system to the peripheral nerves in your legs, arms, shoulders, neck, and core. There, the cells release stored glycogen to fuel chemical reactions and electrolytes like sodium and potassium to spark the electrical impulses that cause your muscle fibers to contract. The result: you tense, turn, coil your legs and midsection, and when the ball arrives—whack! You return the serve with a stinging backhand. All this occurs in a fraction of a second with little or no conscious thought.

With each beat, your heart delivers about three ounces of oxygen-rich blood (2,000 gallons of blood each day) through 60,000 miles of blood vessels and microscopic capillaries that feed every organ, muscle, and bone—as well as the 100-billion-plus neurons in your brain, so you can think clearly. With such a complex dance going on every second of your waking (and sleeping) day, it's easy to understand how much proper cellular function—and, therefore, the proper function of the body's various systems—depends on having the right fuel and raw materials available in plentiful supply.

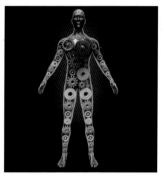

If you fail to give a Ferrari engine (which has only a few thousand moving parts) a single spark plug, it doesn't matter if you have filled it with the finest gasoline and topped off the oil. It won't run right. Imagine what happens when you deny your body, which has trillions of moving parts, the antioxidants it needs to prevent cellular damage or the amino acids it needs to maintain healthy muscle tissue!

The Cell Under Stress

Exercise is stress. When you exercise five or six days per week, you are subjecting your body to a great deal of stress. Now, much of this can be considered "eustress," that is, positive stress that sparks beneficial changes in your tissues. With exercise, you expand the capacity of your cardiovascular system, build muscle strength, burn calories to control your weight and release endorphins to improve your mood—but you already know this. One of the reasons you exercise is because it's one of the most healthful things you can do for your body. But exercise also subjects your body to "distress" that, left unchecked, can cause damage.

When you exercise, your body produces free radicals: unpaired electrons that float around looking to steal electrons from healthy cells. Free radicals cause cellular damage and also damage your DNA. You experience this cellular damage as muscle soreness, inflammation, and injury to soft tissues, joints, connective tissue, or bones. To combat this regular influx of free radicals, your body needs a steady supply of antioxidants, which can only come from your diet. Give your body sufficient nutrients, and you stand a better chance of staying healthy during and after a rough workout. Deny your body what it needs, and you court fatigue, injury, and reduced performance.

This means supplementation. It's simply not practically possible to get all of the complex Power Nutrients you need from eating a healthy, balanced diet that you can manage on a busy schedule. Without dietary supplements, you risk finding yourself mired in the 3D Effect.

Your Cells and the 3D Effect

The athlete's body really is an astonishing example of biological engineering. In part, that's because, even when you are not giving it all the nutrients it needs to repel free radicals, heal tissue damage, and produce sufficient levels of cellular energy, it continues to do those things anyway. If you think about a triathlete at the end of an Ironman™, there's no way he or she can have proper nutrition during the agonizing last miles of a marathon. The triathlete is getting by on will and fitness, and his or her body is paying the price. That's why you see many amateurs and pros in the medical tent at the end of races getting IV electrolytes and carbohydrates. When you push your body too hard without the fuel it needs, there's a price!

You may not be an Ironman™, but you probably want to run faster, jump higher, lift more weight, and have better performance. That means asking more and more of your body. To a point, your body will deliver. But this is the price: when the cells in one system lack sufficient nutrients to meet the demands you're placing on them, they will borrow those nutrients from another system, depleting your body's nutritional stores.

A perfect example of this is what happens when you go on a crash diet. When you shock your body with a radical drop in caloric intake, it goes into starvation mode. Metabolic activity slows down, and your body temperature drops. Your body will also start to burn muscle as fuel. Without enough carbohydrates to power your cells and enough protein to rebuild muscles, you can consume your own healthy tissues, and, in extreme cases, your own organs. This is why fitness trainers counsel their clients on rigorous programs to eat more of the right foods, not less.

Your cells will do their best to respond to the stress you place on them, but the cost is the depletion of important nutrients elsewhere—and **Depletion** is the first part of the 3D Effect. When you continue to make extreme demands of your body without giving it the fuel to meet those demands, you persist in depleting your stores of vital nutrients until you enter the realm of **Deficiency**, where tissues and organs begin to exhibit damage at the cellular level. If this continues, **Dysfunction** can come in the form of chronic injury, weakness, cramping, muscle wasting, or full-blown disease. For example, triathletes commonly suffer from cardiac arrhythmia as a result of the intensity of their sport. In some cases, these faulty heart rhythms have forced athletes to retire and even caused deaths. Though no research into this exists yet, it is likely that this problem stems, in part, from the body's depletion of key nutrients related to cardiac health, such as Coenzyme Q10 and potentially NO.

Simply put, if you are going to stress the body through athletic activity, you must replenish the body through strategic nutrition. And, contrary to popular belief, diet alone just won't get it done.

What Nutrition Means

Most of us, whether we exercise or not, have a nutritionally deficient diet. It's hard to eat healthfully; we get that. While we certainly consume enough calories to keep our bodies going—not getting enough calories is hardly the problem for most Americans—we rarely eat sufficient quantities of fresh, whole, nutrient-rich foods to give us even a basic foundation for wellness.

Many athletes have great diets, and that's laudable. But a healthy diet does not necessarily deliver the nutrients your body needs to compensate for the demands of your sport. The stress of hard workouts and competition means you have greater nutritional needs than the average person, and diet alone won't meet them. Even if you eat an incredibly well-balanced diet, you are probably in a nutrient hole, and in all probability, don't realize the damage you are causing your body.

Do you eat fresh foods in the right balance, complementing your daily intake through supplements? Or, do you spend a few hours sweating it out at the gym and then power down a whey protein shake? Do you skip meals? Do you get the right amount of protein? Are you taking in enough Omega-3 fatty acids? The trouble is, by the time you find out there's a problem, you're regularly experiencing symptoms of **Dysfunction**—the leading edge of a damaging condition you may have had for years and which could take as long to reverse.

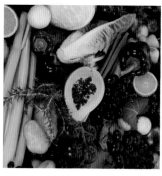

Power Nutrients are not meant to replace good foods, but rather to supplement your diet with the additional nutrients your body needs in the proper doses. You might look and feel fantastic. Maybe you can run for miles and come back for more. But, if you aren't supplementing with the right Power Nutrients, sooner or later there will be a price to pay.

Pay Attention to Your Owner's Manual

It doesn't matter whether you are running three miles a day or training for a marathon. There's a big difference in these two goals, but the nutritional elements your body requires to accomplish them are very similar.

Exercise remains one of the best things you can do for your body. But exercise is intended to enhance the function of every cell in the body. In order to deliver on that functionality, these cells need the right nutrition. Your cells don't care if you are bicycling, swimming, or lifting weights. All they care about is getting the nutrients they need in the right amounts.

Your body puts up with a lot: work, play, exercise, late nights, stress, anger, lack of sleep, unhealthy food, parties, injuries, emotional turmoil, environmental toxins, and a thousand other challenges it faces nearly every day. If your body came with an owner's manual, its page one would tell you to provide it proper fuel and regular maintenance in order to keep it running, maximize its lifespan, and optimize its performance. Consider this book your body's owner's manual for optimal athletic performance. Now, let's talk about nutrients and how they work to power the body's systems.

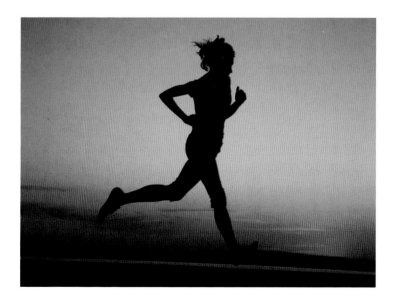

Chapter Two
Nutrition: More Than the Food We Eat

"If we could give every individual the right amount of nourishment and exercise, not too little and not too much, we would have found the safest way to health."

—*Hippocrates*

For anyone, but especially for an athlete, nutrition is about much more than just food intake. You've heard the saying, "Garbage in, garbage out." It's right on target when it comes to the impact of nutrition at the cellular level. The right balance of vital nutrients *biochemically enhances* the function of your cells, which leads to the optimal functioning of your organs and body systems. With poor nutrition—junk food, empty calories, an unbalanced diet—the opposite happens.

If you already follow a healthy dietary regimen, you've made a good start, but it's not enough. Extensive scientific research has shown that many of the amino acids, antioxidants, vitamins, minerals, and proteins that are the foundation for peak performance and health *are simply not available in the foods we eat at levels that deliver the maximum benefits*. In other words, to get some of the **Power Nutrients** you need, in the quantities that will enable your body to operate at its best, you would need to eat massive amounts of food in the right formula at each meal. That's just not practical. First of all, there's the caloric impact. Beyond that, most of us are so busy in our daily lives that our everyday eating habits are questionable at best. But what really makes incomplete nutrition a near emergency for athletes is the stress exercise inflicts on the body.

To Bonk or Not to Bonk?

You've probably bonked before. When you push your body further than its stored energy can handle, it says, "Stop!" There's no more glycogen to fuel the biochemical reactions that power your muscles, and you can't take another step. It's a direct consequence of poor nutrition.

If you find it difficult to increase the amount of weight you lift, get better times in foot or bike races, or seem to run out of gas halfway through a strenuous workout, your cells are trying to tell you something. Your nutrition isn't up to par. A good example is the story of Kevin Everett, a professional triathlete in Boise, Idaho, who has competed in elite endurance races around the world. Kevin relates a story of a 2008 Olympic-length triathlon in Florida when he bonked.

"I was having one of the better races of my life," he says. "I was third or fourth off the bike and was still in the top ten at mile four in the run and was running pretty well. Then, I don't remember anything."

Kevin passed out within sight (1/4 mile or 400 meters) of the finish line. His phosphate levels were completely depleted, and he suffered from a dangerous drop in his cellular oxygen levels.

"I went from having a great race to being passed out on the side of the road," he added. The experience was so frightening it ruined the next several months of his training season.

Kevin is an elite athlete, but like so many, he unknowingly overlooked some of the key nutrients his body needed to meet the demands he was placing on it. As a result, he was not only unable to complete his race but also put his health at risk.

Stress: Good and Bad

Stress gets a bad name…sort of. We think of stress as the result of emotional triggers—like debt, traffic, and busy schedules—that flood our systems with hormones like cortisol and give us headaches and heartburn. But *eustress*, which is defined as "stress that is healthful or giving one the feeling of fulfillment," is a positive thing, especially in athletes.

For example, a *New York Times* article in mid-2010 looked at the correlation between pre-competition stress in swimmers and how these athletes used their anxiety to push themselves to perform better. A physiological adaptation to anxiety diverts blood flow from the digestive system to the muscle during time of stress, providing more oxygen to the muscle in time of need.

Resistance training provides eustress by causing microscopic tears in the muscles used to lift the weight. When the athlete rests after lifting, the repair of that damage is what leads to muscle growth and increased lean body mass. Intense cardiovascular exercise eustresses the heart by forcing it to beat much faster than normal. Over the long term, this strengthens the heart muscle and floods the body with NO, which relaxes and expands the blood vessels, reducing blood pressure and improving cardiovascular health. Exercise helps us burn calories, control weight, and reduce insulin resistance, among many other positives. There are several ways in which exertion-related stress benefits us.

However, when you train intensively for a race, game, or just as part of an ongoing fitness program, you also subject your body to *distress*, or negative stress. This produces many of the same results as the kind of chronic emotional stress that's so common today and so devastating to the body. Your blood pressure soars. Your heart races to 80% or 90% of your maximum. Your digestion slows as your stomach empties of blood so that the muscles can use the oxygen. That's why endurance athletes don't eat much late in races; their impaired digestion produces little extra energy and can cause nausea. Your adrenal glands flood your body with epinephrine (adrenaline) and cortisol.

Most importantly, exercise produces a high level of free radicals within your tissues. Left unchecked, these molecules damage the body at the cellular level, compromising the integrity of cell structures and even harming your DNA, which can lead to cancer and other serious health problems. Antioxidants (which you've surely heard of) "mop up" these stray electrons and prevent them from doing damage. Antioxidants also protect NO and enhance its function, and, as you'll read later, NO is the linchpin of your entire athletic and fitness nutrition program.

The Free Radical Problem

Of course, exercise is usually beneficial. Your body systems all return to normal once the exercise is over, and they can even become healthier over time with regular workouts. But stress is still stress. You are making demands on your body when you exercise: asking your heart to pump faster and more efficiently, your cells to take up stored glucose or fat for energy, and so on. You're damaging your muscles, joints, and connective tissues. You're courting damage from free radicals. Your body needs to recover from the impact of this stress, and doing so requires sufficient nutrients in the right proportions. Having a high-protein shake and a salad after your 75-minute, high-intensity interval training session is a good start, but nutritionally, in the long term, that just isn't going to get it done.

The more intensely and frequently you exercise, the more you need antioxidants in abundance to counteract free radical activity. But you won't get enough, even with the healthiest dietary program. Even if you're an elite athlete with a fantastic diet, if you get no supplemental nutrition, you will eventually experience performance plateaus or become injured.

Antioxidant neutralizing a free radical

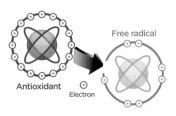

Antioxidant nutrients protect the body by neutralizing free radicals.

If you're putting athletic demands on your body, but also struggling with a so-so diet, the depletion of key nutrients will occur faster and the consequences—acute injury, poor recovery, chronic health conditions—will appear faster and likely be more severe. You will quickly move from **Depletion** to **Deficiency** to **Dysfunction**.

In athletes, the **3D Effect** is the body's response to exercise-related stress, combined with inadequate nutrition. As an athlete, you're stressing your body in ways that can be healthy, but only when you give your physiology what it needs to perform, heal, and recover. That means supplementation. It's pure logic:

If all cell function depends on nutrition, and exercise is a stress, which over time, depletes the body of nutrition, then athletes must supplement to perform optimally.

Supplements: A Complement to Diet

Supplements are not food. They are in a nutritional class all by themselves. Unlike the carbohydrates, fats, and proteins you consume in food, supplements generally do not provide you with calories. That's not their job. They are substances that the body uses to spark specific biochemical reactions within the cells that produce beneficial effects in your body. Think of them as the oil, coolant, and hydraulic fluid that you put in your car. They don't provide the energy to make your engine run, but they do make it possible for your engine to run more efficiently, safely, and productively. Without them, your car would be basically useless.

It's time to stop thinking of supplements as optional adjuncts to our normal diet and start thinking of them as an essential part of an athlete's core nutritional program! The right supplementation regimen will enhance any diet and exercise program. If you engage in extreme exercise on a regular basis, either as a professional or high-level recreational athlete or fitness professional, then supplementation is a crucial complement to an already optimal dietary regimen.

As a central part of your foundational nutrition strategy, a supplementation program that's optimized for your unique biochemistry will give you more energy during the day, power you through your fitness routine, and help you recover more fully. It will also deliver more NO to your tissues, which will supercharge your performance, as well as enhance your overall wellness.

You Have the Power

Do you want to improve your exercise performance, strengthen your heart, fight disease, and reduce your recovery time? You can. There is not one specific eating plan or exercise program that you need to follow in order to achieve this. However, you should be aware of your personal eating habits and nutritional intake and make an effort to adjust them if they are less than optimal. Ask yourself:

- **Do I skip meals?** If so, make a point to eat at least three meals a day. Even better, eat five to six smaller meals, with a balance of complex carbohydrates, lean proteins, and healthy fats, to provide a consistent flow of nutrients and maintain a high metabolism.

- **Do I eat fresh vegetables, fruits, nuts, seeds, whole grains, and lean proteins in adequate quantities?** Throughout the day, these foods should comprise most of your food intake. Watch your protein intake; the more punishing your sport or workout, the more protein you need to fuel recovery.

- **Do I drink at least 8 -12 8 ounce glasses of water a day if I am exercising?** Hydration improves digestion, muscle repair and athletic performance. It helps regulate your body temperature. To increase nutrient delivery and uptake, you need more water.

- **Do I eat too much fat, sugar, and starch or take in too many empty calories?** If so, think about replacing them with healthy alternatives like fruits and whole grains.

- **Am I supplementing my diet with quality nutritional supplements that help my body produce more NO?** This is your key to increasing your exercise performance!

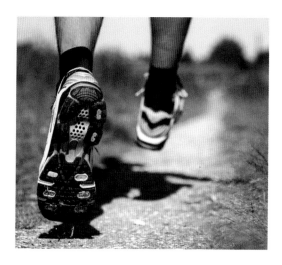

Chapter Three
Nitric Oxide: The Hidden Benefit of Exercise

Nitric oxide, or NO, is the natural performance booster that strengthens your heart, lungs, and nerves, along with every cell in your body. It also allows you to prolong your exercise, and prolonged exercise increases NO levels in the body. It's a virtuous cycle that can lead to improved athletic performance and better health.

You may not have heard about NO from the media or fitness or nutritional professionals, and your personal physician may not even know much about it, but biochemists and physiologists have known about its effects for years. Now, an increasing body of rigorous research is revealing that NO may be the single most important nutrient for promoting optimal cellular function, athletic performance, health, and wellness in the human body. In 1998, the Nobel Committee deemed the research regarding NO to be so important that they awarded the Nobel Prize in Medicine to Dr. Ignarro and two other scientists.

In medical terms, NO is a short-lived, gaseous molecule that is produced in your cells. Once released into the bloodstream, it signals the body to perform certain functions such as vasodilation opening up the blood vessels and capillaries to increase blood flow and deliver oxygen and critical nutrients throughout your body at the time it needs them most. Do you ever wonder why people suffering from chest pain are often prescribed and instructed to take nitroglycerine? It's because the body uses nitroglycerine to produce high levels of NO quickly by opening the coronary arteries and increasing the flow of blood to the heart.

For the athlete seeking enhanced performance, endurance and strength, as well as faster recovery, the availability of NO in the body is critically important. As any endurance athlete can tell you, a triathlon or other long-distance event becomes a competition between body parts over demand for the blood supply. The skin wants the blood circulating to dissipate heat, but the muscles are screaming for the oxygen and nutrients that the blood carries. Meanwhile, the

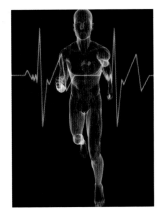

stomach needs blood to digest food and make those nutrients available in the first place. It's not hard to see how ample NO, with its ability to increase circulation, would be critical to athletic performance.

But as additional research is beginning to show us, NO doesn't stop with cardiovascular benefits. It now appears that NO is the "master signaling molecule" throughout the body, and that maintaining sufficient levels through exercise and nutrition not only improves cardiovascular condition but also optimizes the function of every body system; this leads to superior athletic results and greater wellness, quality of life, and even longevity.

What NO Is

When you exercise, your body goes through a remarkable process during which it releases NO into your bloodstream. As stated earlier, NO is a "signaling molecule." Its sole function is to send out various biological signals that regulate the activity of cells and instruct the body to perform certain functions. Some of the benefits that your body gains from NO include increased blood flow to muscles and organs as well as better cardiovascular and enhanced lung functions, but that's just the tip of the proverbial iceberg. It turns out that NO benefits nearly every cell and system in the body.

NO is primarily manufactured in the *endothelium*, which is the layer of cells lining the interior surface of the blood vessels. The endothelial tissue, which separates the blood from the smooth muscles of the vessel walls, is extremely thin and fragile. Remember earlier, when we told you that there are approximately six trillion endothelial cells in the average human body? It's easy to see what occurs when such a vast, crucial cellular network gets what it needs to function at its biological peak. When your endothelium is well nourished, it produces NO at optimal levels. The NO then rapidly spreads through the cell membranes to the underlying muscle cells, causing the arteries to dilate and blood to flow unimpeded to the heart and other organs.

NO is also produced in the nerve cells and controls many functions, such as the workings of your gastrointestinal system. When NO is produced in white blood cells, it can be used to kill invading bacteria and parasites.

What NO Does

Because NO functions on a localized basis, it is released by billions of cells throughout the body, enhancing overall functioning. The longer NO circulates in the body, the greater benefit it provides to your cells, cardiovascular system, lungs, nervous system, and organs and the more optimal their functionality will be. The more efficiently each of your cells function, the more you will be able to produce peak speed, strength, and endurance as part of your athletic endeavors.

Also, the desirable effects of NO aren't limited to athletes. On the contrary, this molecule is quickly becoming regarded as a critical component of a pro-wellness lifestyle for all people, ranging from athletes to the sedentary. Some of the benefits of sufficient levels of NO include:

- Helping to increase cardiovascular capacity and circulation and enhancing oxygen and nutrient delivery to cells.

- Helping cells get rid of waste products.

- Regulating the muscle tone of blood vessels and having a major impact in controlling blood pressure.

- Stopping blood platelets from forming clots, which helps prevent arterial blockages and heart attacks.

- Transmitting messages between nerve cells, a process known as neurotransmission.

NO helps slow the accumulation of *atherosclerotic plaque* in the blood vessels. This artery hardening build up of cholesterol and fats that narrow or block the arteries is a major precursor to coronary heart disease, leading to heart attack and stroke. Our research strongly suggests that NO's ability to combat this plaque helps produce healthy levels of cholesterol by working in concert with medications commonly prescribed for people with high cholesterol.

NO also helps the immune system fight bacterial infections, viruses, and parasites, and even decreases the growth of certain types of cancer. NO is crucial to memory function, as the brain uses it to help neurons store and retrieve long-term memories and transmit information. As an anti-inflammatory agent, NO is being studied for its potential role in reducing the swelling and discomfort of osteoarthritis and rheumatoid arthritis.

Where NO Comes From and How to Make It

It is not yet known how much NO is normally present in the body or what levels are optimal. This gas is difficult to measure, because it disappears almost instantly upon exposure to air. But we do know that, beginning in early adulthood, NO levels gradually decline, probably due to damage to the endothelial cells caused by factors such as stress, a high-fat diet, and a sedentary lifestyle.

Consequently, few people produce enough NO to keep their cardiovascular systems functioning smoothly. As we age, certain metabolic conditions can lead to a depletion of NO in our bodies, allowing the molecule to fall below optimal levels. We under produce NO when endothelial tissue is damaged by age, illness, a toxic environment, or genetic predisposition, at which point we become vulnerable to disease. Stress, high levels of free radicals, a sedentary lifestyle, and a poor diet also reduce NO levels. That's a problem, because the benefits of NO—from increased heart health, to fighting infection and disease to decreasing the risk of developing type 2 diabetes—are clear and backed by scientific research. Again, Dr. Ignarro won his Nobel Prize specifically for his groundbreaking discoveries about the benefits of NO.

Thus, it is in everyone's interest to optimize the body's production and stores of this miraculous molecule. There are two ways to achieve this: exercise and nutrition. In essence:

Exercise + Nutritional Supplementation = Nitric Oxide (NO) Production

Exercise alone increases NO production threefold to fourfold. The more you exercise, the more NO you create. That may be the source of much of the systemic—or body-wide—health benefits of exercise. Yes, the most important long-term benefit of exercise may be the chronic elevation of NO and the positive downstream effects it creates. Once your body produces NO, other Power

Nutrients such as antioxidants, L-glutamine, Coenzyme Q10, and essential fatty acids protect it from free radical damage and ensure that it is used with the greatest efficiency and effectiveness by the systems in which it is needed.

Regular exercise, and a regular infusion of nutrients via diet and supplementation, works synergistically to give your body everything it needs to produce and maintain optimal levels of NO in your tissues. Just 20 minutes of aerobic exercise three times a week will optimize your NO production, although, if you are an athlete, you are probably already exercising far beyond those minimal levels. But, even if you are only spending one hour a week in an activity that raises your heart rate, you are already boosting your NO levels.

We have also discovered new nutritional strategies that athletes and non-athletes alike can use to increase NO production. Our bodies can synthesize NO from the amino acid L-arginine, which is found in protein-rich foods and used by every cell in your body. Studies have shown that L-arginine is a major precursor of NO in the body and that increasing L-arginine intake increases the production of NO. For this reason, L-arginine is one of the key Power Nutrients that we recommend.

Since L-arginine is present in dietary protein, wouldn't just eating a lot more protein provide you with what you need? Not really. To ingest L-arginine in the amount necessary to boost NO production, you would have to eat large quantities of meat and other high-protein foods. That's not easy, especially if you're working out and trying to maintain a competition weight. Also, L-arginine tends to be most *bioavailable*—that is, most accessible to the cells—when taken along with the amino acid L-citrulline. The complexity of proper

**Nitric Oxide
Increases Blood Flow**

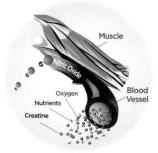

*By increasing blood flow, Nitric Oxide
supports the delivery of oxygen and nutrients
(like creatine) to the muscle.*

NO nutrition is why supplementation is an irreplaceable component of your performance plan.

Taking quality dietary and nutritional supplements—including antioxidants like Vitamins C and E and Selenium—formulated to the correct potency provides your body with the elements that produce and maintain healthy NO levels, thus increasing its beneficial properties. This is why exercise, diet, and supplementation must all be a part of the daily regimen of any athlete who is serious about getting peak performance out of his or her marvelous machine.

NO and Performance

With that, let's talk about NO and athletic performance. An increased supply of NO in your body accelerates the expansion of blood vessels and produces enhanced blood flow throughout your body, which means faster and more effective delivery of nutrients like amino acids, glucose, and oxygen to the muscle fibers. This helps your muscles work more efficiently and recover faster while facilitating the removal of waste products like lactic acid and carbon dioxide that can decrease performance.

As your exercise level increases, so, too, does the demand for nutrition. Your body calls for more NO, but if you don't have the nutritional foundation to enable your body to make as much of the molecule as it needs, you won't have what it takes to meet the demand when the time comes. This can be the difference between winning a race and not being able to finish it, or between hauling yourself up that last hold on the rock face and giving up from exhaustion.

Research shows that taking NO-promoting nutrients in coordination with a NO-friendly diet and regular fitness training results in faster run and cycling times, less fatigue, and quicker recovery after a workout or injury. For example, Coenzyme Q10 boosts cellular energy production as well as protects the cardiac muscle. Omega-3 fatty acids, such as those found in fish oil, help maintain healthy cell membrane structure and function and also promote healthy heart rhythm, something that's important to endurance athletes who pend many hours on a racecourse. Glucosamine promotes joint health, aiding in injury prevention, thus enhancing exercise performance. Vitamin D offers a host of benefits that we're still learning about, from better cognitive health to boosted immune health. To learn more about the benefits of Glucosamine and Vitamin D, refer to the book *Health is Wealth: 10 Power Nutrients That Increase Your Odds of Living to 100 (Heath Value Publications 2009)* or visit www.HealthisWealth.net.

Taken together, Power Nutrients boost the well-being and function of the *entire* athlete.

Think about your exercise routine. Whether lifting weights, running, cycling, swimming, or playing team sports is your thing, your muscles need nutrients and oxygen to keep pumping and working harder. That means a generous blood supply. Imagine what would happen if you were in the middle of bench-pressing 250 lbs. when your blood flow was suddenly cut in half. The results would be ugly.

You won't have to worry about this as you work your upper body, as long as the cells in your blood vessels release NO, which signals your arteries and veins to either dilate or constrict in order to send blood and nutrients where they are needed at that moment. In this way, NO helps regulate your ability to perform strenuous exercise, as well as gives you the potential, with proper fuel from healthy food, to tap into higher levels of performance on demand.

For the serious athlete, but also for the weekend athlete, gym rat, or workplace softball player, NO is the key to getting the full benefits from workouts, preventing injury, and "bringing it" when the pressure is on, whether that means the bike stage of a triathlon, the fourth quarter of a basketball game, or the end of a long, tiring martial arts class. It's a yin and yang relationship: exercise and nutrition help keep NO at optimal levels in your body, and in return, NO nourishes your body and enables you to keep exercising and producing more and more NO. If you embrace the power of supplements as part of a holistic and complete nutritional solution, you'll be one step closer to getting the performance out of your body that you desire.

Being an "athlete" is only one way to describe you. You're also a person who craves vibrant health and a long, happy life. Well, NO and exercise can be the difference makers there as well. Let's explore how.

> *"So many people spend their health gaining wealth, and then have to spend their wealth to regain their health."*
>
> – *A.J. Reb Materi*

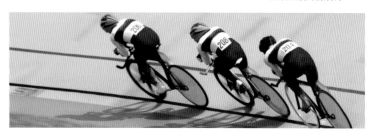

Chapter Four

The Benefits of Exercise: Health Equals Wealth

"Movement is a medicine for creating change in a person's physical, emotional, and mental states."
—*Carol Welch*

Why is exercise good for us? The message that exercise is beneficial is everywhere, but why is it such a potent tool for promoting not just excellent athletic performance but also health, longevity, and quality of life? Yes, resistance training leads to bigger muscles and greater lean body mass. Yes, regular exercise increases metabolism, burns more calories, and helps us maintain a healthy weight. But it seems that exercise does much, much more than that. Why?

In this chapter, we'll look at the mechanism that underlies the incredible health benefits of exercise and how exercise, combined with a quality diet and supplementation, can make vital deposits in our biological bank account, increasing our odds of a long, active, athletic, prosperous, and enjoyable life.

How Exercise Changes the Body

You're an athlete, so you know more about the positive impact of exercise than the average person. Depending on the kind of workouts and sports you do, you might enjoy more speed and endurance, superior strength, improved mood, a lean and muscular body, or a sharper mental state than people who are relatively sedentary. But the wonders of exercise are not limited to athletes. Even if you have incorporated movement into your life through walking, climbing stairs, and doing yard work, you're getting health benefits, though they may not be as obvious.

Here's a comprehensive list of the positive impact regular exercise can have on your body, depending on the kind, duration, intensity, and regularity of your workouts:

Why Is Exercise Good for Us?

- Higher nitric oxide levels
- Increased heart rate—improves the heart's ability to contract during exercise
- Improved circulation
- Reduced blood pressure
- Increased muscle strength and flexibility
- Improved insulin utilization—reduces type 2 diabetes risk
- Increased muscle tone
- Higher lean body mass and better weight control
- Increased energy
- Increased HDL ("good") cholesterol
- Improved digestion and elimination
- Reduced incidence of depression
- Improved sexual performance
- Enhanced mood
- Delay or prevention of cellular aging
- Prevention of many forms of cancer
- Greater joint mobility and lubrication—reduces risk of osteoarthritis
- Increased respiratory capacity and cardiovascular endurance
- Improved neuromuscular coordination and balance
- Enhanced immune system and disease resistance
- Improved flexibility and core strength
- Enhanced body power and speed
- Stronger bones and reduced osteoporosis risk
- Reduced stress levels
- Improved concentration and mental function
- Better sleep
- Reduced anxiety
- Feelings of well-being

Source: *The Guidelines For Exercise Testing And Prescription* by the American College of Sports Medicine.

Exercise reduces the risk factors for heart disease, diabetes, osteoporosis, and even depression. It is proven to increase longevity and improve quality of life. Many of these incredible improvements are due, in great part, to the action of NO. For years, scientists, fitness professionals, and athletes alike knew that exercise produced an abundance of positive changes in physiology, but they didn't really understand why. Is it all about weight loss? Exercise improves cardiovascular function and blood pressure, but how?

With more intensive research into NO, we have the answers. This molecule, when increased by exercise and diet, increases circulation and improves the health of the heart and blood vessels. It enhances the transmission of nerve signals and improves mood. It optimizes the effectiveness of the immune system at fighting off disease. It activates the body's anti-inflammatory mechanisms, helping prevent arthritis and also reducing inflammation in arteries, which is thought to be a major risk factor for heart attack and stroke. It's a big part of the reason that exercising not only makes you look and move better, but also makes you feel better and healthier.

While exercise delivers some of its powerful plusses by boosting the metabolic rate, building muscle, increasing mobility, and enhancing flexibility, many of the signal benefits we talk about are largely due to the abundance of NO the body experiences when strenuous exercise is fueled by complete, supplemented nutrition.

Specific Exercise Benefits

We can lump exercise into three broad categories: strength training (weightlifting, core training), cardiovascular conditioning (running, cycling, aerobics), and flexibility training (yoga, stretching). As an athlete, you probably participate in all three. Let's look at the specific ways in which each promotes optimal health and function:

Strength Training
- *Maintains strength and power*
- *Increases lean body mass*
- *Greater core strength prevents back problems*
- *Boosts metabolic rate by up to 15%, aiding in weight control*
- *Prevents osteoporosis*
- *Increases ligament tensile strength*
- *Increases tendon tensile strength*

Cardiovascular Conditioning
- Increases oxygen intake
- Increases the body's oxygen use efficiency
- Increases cardiac output and efficiency
- Increases blood volume
- Improves stamina
- Improves lung health and capacity
- Reduces blood pressure and lowers resting heart rate
- Improves cholesterol ratio (HDL/LDL)
- Increases insulin sensitivity
- Improves circulation to active muscles
- Decreases symptoms of anxiety and depression

Flexibility Training
- Improves range of motion
- Reduces risk of injury
- Reduces post-workout soreness
- Improves posture
- Improves circulation to muscles
- Enhances neuromuscular coordination
- Improves balance

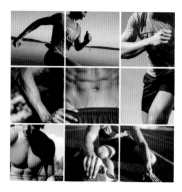

In short, within these three major subcategories of exercise, in all their infinite varieties of moves, machines, plusses, and routines, you have the secrets to maximum health for every system of the body, down to the cellular level. Exercise is not only the key to peak athletic performance, but also the fountain of youth. That is, if you keep giving your body what it needs.

Even Athletes Age

As an athlete, you are not the average American. You're probably in better shape than 90% of the people around you. But do you intend to continue your exercise regimen throughout your life? Even athletes age, get sick, and experience disease. But, by continuing your healthy exercise and dietary habits throughout your life, you dramatically increase your odds of enjoying years, or even decades, of healthy, active living.

Also, by reducing your need for costly healthcare as you age, regular exercise (along with proper nutrition) can save you tens or even hundreds of thousands of dollars. As we detailed in *Health Is Wealth*, preventive lifestyle choices like regular exercise can prevent some of the most financially costly medical interventions from ever becoming necessary. How much money would you save by never needing a coronary bypass, knee replacement, costly statin drugs, angioplasty, or prescription antidepressants? Health really does equal wealth!

Athlete-Specific Physiological Benefits of Regular Exercise

1. Adaptive physiologic response increases
2. Aerobic work capacity increases
3. Body fat stores drop
4. Capillary density and blood flow to active muscles increases
5. Resting heart rate is reduced
6. Vascular return increases
7. Lactate threshold increases
8. Lung diffusion capacity increases
9. Maximum ventilation increases
10. Maximum cardiac output increases
11. Maximum oxygen consumption increases
12. Mobilization and utilization of stored fat increases

Source: *The Guidelines For Exercise Testing And Prescription* by the American College Of Sports Medicine.

However, enjoying all of the long-term wellness benefits of rigorous exercise into your seventies, eighties, and beyond is probably not possible, unless you give your body what it needs to repair and heal itself through a lifetime of correct nutrition. The stresses of years of vigorous strength training and aerobic conditioning can deplete cellular levels of critical nutrients, leading to the 3D Effect and Dysfunction in the body's systems. Poor nutrition can turn the positives of exercise into negatives: stress fractures, cardiac arrhythmias, strains, sprains, and more. To prevent this and be able to continue to exercise regularly, you need to make Power Nutrients a regular part of your nutritional regimen… permanently.

BioDebt and BioWealth

Making regular deposits into your body's account of essential nutrients helps you stave off disease, or what we call **BioDebt**. We developed this concept in our last book because, from the perspective of nutrient-based, natural medical science, what we think of as disease is really the end-stage dysfunction that occurs after certain body systems are depleted of vital nutrients over a long period of time. Through poor diet, stress, sedentary lifestyle, pollution, cigarette smoking, and other causes, many Americans spend decades depleting their stores of critical antioxidants, vitamins, minerals, and phytochemicals. After Depletion becomes Deficiency, systems begin to malfunction. Eventually, those malfunctions become substantial enough that we experience them as symptoms: chest pain, fatigue, fractures, joint pain, insomnia, etc.

When you have drawn on your body's account of Power Nutrients for so long (without replenishing it) that your balance is close to zero, you are in **BioDebt**. We feel that's a more accurate name for disease, because it reflects the true cause of most disease: a chronic, long-term deficiency of key nutrients, leading to biological dysfunction. That's why we call vascular disease *endothelial dysfunction*; it's the arterial lining or endothelium that's not functioning optimally, leaving the arteries constricted, inflamed, and clogged with plaque. Obesity becomes *metabolic dysfunction*, depression becomes *neurochemical dysfunction*, and so on.

As an athlete, you may be in better health today than your non-athletic peers. But you are also asking more of your body—drawing more from your bank account of critical nutrients. If that account is not replenished steadily over the years, you become far more likely to go into **BioDebt**, despite your high level of fitness. Remember, exercise and nutrition—diet and supplementation— complement one another. The more you withdraw via athletic training and sports, the more you need to deposit via the plate, shake, and capsule.

Like financial debt, **BioDebt** can sometimes be reversed, but the longer the deficiency has gone on, the longer it takes for an infusion of nutrients to reverse the cellular damage that has accumulated over the years. Sometimes, the damage is irreversible. All the Coenzyme Q10 in the world will do only so much to rehabilitate heart muscle devastated by years of neglect, obesity, and diabetes.

As you age, with the desire to remain active and fit, it's much better to achieve the state we call BioWealth. As you can guess, this is the opposite of **BioDebt** and is our term for whole-body wellness and well-being. When you are in BioWealth, you are constantly making deposits of Power Nutrients into your biological account via diet and supplements, in addition to enjoying the broad array of benefits conferred by regular exercise. With a sufficient supply of vital chemicals, your cells can function optimally, giving you what you need to get peak performance, but also maintaining long-term cellular health.

Attaining a state of BioWealth is about *preventing* disease and disability from ever occurring. It's about a holistic state of prime function, where each cell in each system has what it needs to operate at its peak for as long as possible. Athletes in a state of BioWealth not only perform better when they are in their competitive prime, but can continue to engage in their sports for decades, long after many Americans have resigned themselves to life on the couch or in the doctor's office. You know those eighty-year-olds you see doing Ironman™ triathlons and sporting cut pectorals and quads? You can bet they are BioWealthy.

Built to Move

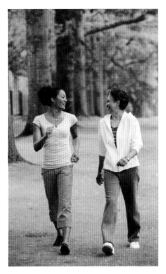

A study by the Department of Nutrition at the Harvard School of Public Health and Brigham and Women's Hospital followed 115,000 women over a 24-year period to determine how a person's level of physical activity and body fat could be predictors for premature death. Researchers found that a high level of physical activity did not eliminate the risk of premature death associated with obesity, and being lean did not eliminate the risk in mortality associated with inactivity. In other words, **longevity means being both active *and* lean.**

Frank Hu, the study's lead author and an associate professor of nutrition and epidemiology at the Harvard School of Public Health, notes that people should be as active as possible, no matter what their weight. It is equally important, however, to maintain a healthy weight and prevent weight gain through diet and lifestyle.

We were built to move. Being sedentary promotes **BioDebt**. A study done by University Medical Center in Rotterdam and published in the *Archives of Internal Medicine* revealed that a daily workout could add nearly four years to the typical life span. That's great news for athletes, who already engage in daily, or near-daily, fitness programs.

In part by increasing levels of NO, which improves immune function and reduces inflammation, exercise also plays a powerful role in preventing disease conditions from developing. Check out these incredible statistics:

- More than 60 studies suggest that women who exercise regularly can expect a 20%-30% reduction in the chance of developing breast cancer, as compared with women who don't exercise.

- Colorectal cancer has been one of the most extensively studied cancers in relation to physical activity, with more than 50 studies examining this association. Many of them have consistently found that adults who increase their physical activity can reduce their risk of developing colon cancer by 30%-40%—relative to those who are sedentary—regardless of body mass index.

- At least 21 studies have examined the impact of physical activity on the risk of lung cancer. Overall, these studies suggest an inverse association between physical activity and lung cancer risk, with the most physically active individuals experiencing about a 20% reduction in risk.

Exercise may also help prevent the aging process at the cellular level. Nobel Prize winning research has found, for the first time, that exercise appears to slow the degeneration of the *telomeres* that are part of each chromosome. Telomeres are sequences of DNA that determine how many times a given cell can divide. Each time a cell reproduces—in building new muscle tissue, for example—the telomere gets a little shorter. When it reaches its end, the cell can no longer divide and some genetic information is lost. Eventually, tissues can no longer repair and renew themselves; as a result breakdown and disease ensue. Researchers now believe that telomere degeneration may be a primary cause of aging.

It appears that exercise may protect the body against the aging process. Studies show that people who exercise most have telomeres that appear to be from five to nine years younger than those who exercise the least. So, it's possible that exercise may not only help you feel and act younger, but can actually make you biologically younger as well.

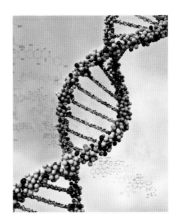

Health Increases Your Wealth

As we've shown you, there are many good reasons to maintain your rigorous athletic activity. However, to do so for decades requires that you fuel your body properly with Power Nutrients. Every time you move your muscles, critical nutrients and reparative enzymes flood your bloodstream to help combat the ongoing damage done to cells, tissues, and organs. Your immune system, cardiovascular system, and nervous system benefit from these nutrients on a microscopic level. You must feed these cellular systems to replace what they lose in repair and recovery.

One of the reasons we often hear from athletes and non-athletes alike as to why they don't take dietary supplements is that they are expensive. It's true that high quality formulations of Power Nutrients, with safeguards for purity and potency, are not cheap. However, they are far less costly than today's most common medical interventions.

As an athlete seeking lifelong activity and productivity from your body, the final benefit of optimal nutrition is *wealth*. Fueling your body properly for the stress of athletic activity not only increases your BioWealth by preventing disease and disability, it also increases your financial wealth. In a time when healthcare costs are rising at a rate far exceeding that of inflation, reducing or eliminating many of the healthcare costs often associated with aging can make you more fiscally fit as well.

We go into great detail about this issue in our previous book, *Health is Wealth*, but it bears repeating from the perspective of an athlete. It doesn't take much imagination to see why saving the $50,000 cost of a coronary bypass is a good thing. But the savings of the Power Nutrient strategy go much further. Consider a more common athletic injury. Suppose that you are a distance runner. After years of running marathons and triathlons, during which you did not give your body the proper quantities of Power Nutrients it required, your knees are shot. Your ligaments are frayed and osteoarthritis (or, as we call it, *connective tissue dysfunction*) leaves you in constant pain. So, you have both knees replaced. Problem solved, right?

Not necessarily. According to CostHelper.com, a Medicare patient undergoing a knee replacement at Dartmouth-Hitchcock Medical Center in Lebanon, New Hampshire, can expect to pay $4,257 out-of-pocket for a knee replacement, including deductibles and coinsurance. That's per knee. So, if you have both knees done, you're out nearly $9,000. Then, there's the cost of pain medication, physical therapy, lost work income if you're employed, and possible home care. You might be out $15,000—or more, if you're not old enough for Medicare and have high-deductible insurance.

Multiply that expense by ten and you get what the typical, out-of-shape American might spend after age forty on healthcare services that could be largely prevented by avoiding nutritional deficiency and engaging in regular exercise. What could you do with $150,000 more in your bank account? Maintaining optimal nutrient levels and engaging in regular, strenuous exercise can save you money on direct healthcare costs, but it can also reduce or eliminate prescription drug costs, insurance premiums, rehabilitation expenses, lost wages, specialized equipment, and more. Avoiding **BioDebt** also reduces the incredible stress on you and your family that comes with health problems.

Imagine more peace of mind, more years of vibrant athletic activity, a fantastic quality of life, *and* greater financial security. That's real wealth.

You now understand the fundamental facts about the links between exercise, diet, nutritional supplements, NO, and money. They will provide an excellent jumping-off point for Part II of the book, where we will look at the impact of supplementation and NO on specific sports and athletes.

> *"Physical fitness can neither be achieved by wishful thinking nor outright purchase."*
>
> —Joseph Pilates

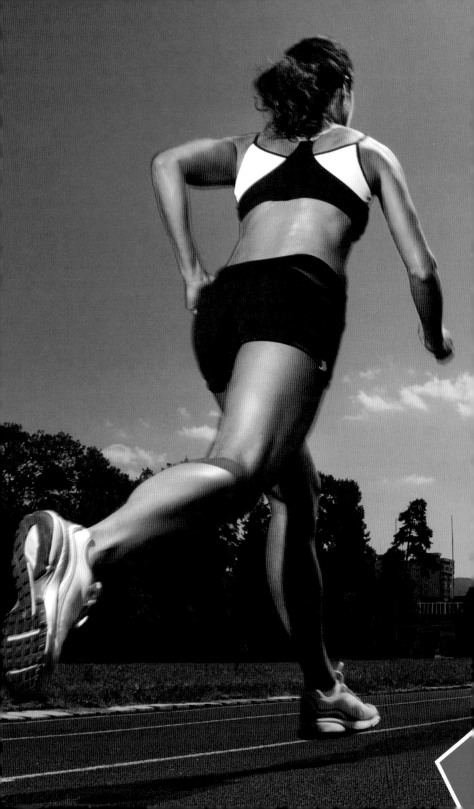

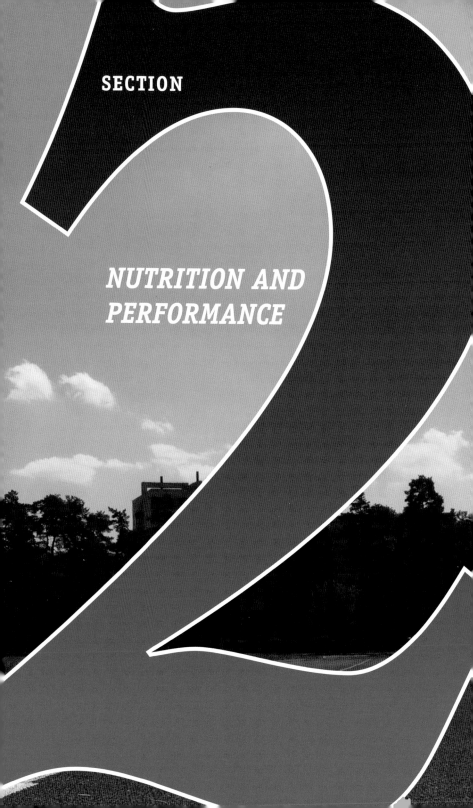

SECTION

2

NUTRITION AND PERFORMANCE

Nutrition and Performance

What we are finding as we speak to more athletes and trainers is that they don't know what they don't know. Surprisingly few athletes, including elite professionals, take some or any dietary supplements as part of their training regimen. The reason for this is simple ignorance. The information on the marvelous benefits of Power Nutrient supplementation is not reaching these athletes or their support teams through the normal media channels, just as it's not reaching the average weekend athlete. That makes *Health Is Wealth: Performance Nutrition* that much more important.

In this section, we will attempt to cure this ignorance by breaking down how nutrition—and, more specifically, key Power Nutrients—impacts performance in the four critical areas of athletic activity: speed, strength, endurance, and recovery. As part of these next four chapters, we interview several top athletes, in a variety of disciplines, about their exercise and nutritional programs. You will note that few of them supplement substantially, and only one uses NO to promote nutrition.

This not only serves to underscore the general lack of awareness of NO, but to highlight an important point: because of their extraordinary levels of physical activity, their bodies are awash in NO. This is surely one of the reasons behind their exceptional athletic results. Yet, because they do not supplement, they are missing out on the Power Nutrients' ability to prevent the stress-related damage of exercise and boost their NO levels even higher. How much *more* could they achieve with supplementation? We will find out.

Chapter Five
Nutrition and Speed

Sprinters. Short-course triathletes. Speed skaters. Base stealers in baseball. Football wide receivers. Soccer strikers. For all these athletes, speed plays a pivotal role. Athletes who rely on speed ask their bodies to deliver explosive performance in short bursts designed to propel them forward on the playing field faster than their opponents. And while the conventional wisdom says, "You can't teach speed," it is possible to train and fuel the body to bring out its optimal speed, regardless of the sport.

Athletic speed arises from the performance of the so-called "fast-twitch" muscle fibers. These muscle fibers can contract quickly and with greater force than the blood-rich "slow-twitch" muscles, but these movements can only be sustained for a short time before they become painful. Speed-centric athletes train specifically for speed, forcing the muscles to work to decrease contraction time, improve "turnover" (the time it takes to move one limb through a motion such as a stride or swim stroke and start the other limb on that same motion), and optimize the neural networks and motor pathways that carry the contraction signals to the muscles.

Several types of movement fit under the umbrella term "speed":

- **Quickness**—This is usually regarded as "first step" acceleration. In other words, how fast can an athlete go from being relatively motionless to at or near top velocity, especially in comparison to an opponent? The most common examples here would be a first-step dribble in man-to-man defense in basketball, a wide receiver running to get open in football, and a base stealer sprinting to the base in baseball. In all cases, quickness is more important than raw speed, because what beats the opponent is nearly immediate acceleration.

- **Explosiveness**—This is the fast application of muscular power; it can be thought of as "speed meets strength." Jumping, in many forms, is probably the most familiar type of explosiveness: a basketball player rising for a dunk, a gymnast doing a floor exercise, or a boxer unleashing a lightning-fast combination of devastating punches.

- **Sustained or Linear Speed**—This is the type of speed most people think about when they hear the word—speed in a line, such as on a running course. This kind of speed might have to be sustained for several minutes if the athlete is engaged in something like a one-mile race or a goal-to-goal run on the soccer field. Fast turnover of the legs is vital to sustained speed.

- **Agility**—This is speed applied to non-linear movement, the ability to quickly contort the body to move laterally as well as vertically. Agility also involves such qualities as flexibility and strength, but, in an athletic setting, it demands speed first and foremost. Examples include mogul skiers, soccer players, and football running backs, all of whom must change direction with lightning speed during the course of their sports.

As we have seen and discussed, vital nutrients play a critical role in the health and performance of the nervous and muscular systems. Thus, they also impact the development and maintenance of athletic speed. Maintaining sufficient stores of needed nutrients at the cellular level enables your body to respond to the demand for speed. Muscles can contract more powerfully to

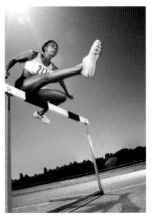

provide explosiveness. Nerve impulses reach muscles more quickly to direct the body through agility moves. The mitochondria in the cells manufacture the additional energy necessary for quick "first step" action, whether playing in a pickup basketball game or diving for a shot as a soccer goalie. Muscles gain the ability to maintain speed longer during the anaerobic activity of sustained running or cycling, allowing you to sprint on the track or pass other cyclists on the triathlon course.

Each of these functions of speed is dependent on proper training, sufficient rest, and supplementation and nutrition during competition, as well as a steady influx of vital nutrients. However, we will focus on the two main sources of long-term nutrients: a balanced, healthy diet and dietary supplementation with Power Nutrients.

NO and Speed

As it is for most of the body's systems, nitric oxide (NO) is a critical element in producing athletic speed. NO controls the vascular tree that directs blood flow to the areas of the body screaming for oxygen and nutrients during a sprint or other speed-based activity (e.g., the lungs, large muscles like the quadriceps, etc.). By controlling the dilation of blood vessels, NO also regulates blood pressure as the body changes position, such as in a 50-meter swim or a hurdles race. This helps to maintain blood flow to the brain and other critical areas of function that are affected by dynamic movements of the body.

When a runner, or other speed athlete, engages the anaerobic system and the mitochondrial energy sources that power muscles during the fast movements of a sprint or cycling race, NO optimizes the transport of glucose to working muscles. By allowing blood to flow more freely, NO enables critical systems to receive energy, shed heat, and get the oxygen they desperately need.

Sufficient levels of NO are therefore critical for optimal speed, and, as they cannot come from exercise if the athlete lacks the energy, oxygen, or circulatory volume to engage in intense work, NO promotion must come from diet and supplements. Proper supplementation with Power Nutrients is the key to unlocking the potential of NO, which, in turn, unlocks the maximum energy contained in the food you consume and the oxygen you breathe.

Eating for Speed

Apart from the specific benefits of certain foods for runners and other athletes, speed requires a high level of quality carbohydrates. Simply put, speed demands energy. Unlike endurance sports, where a lower heart rate can put you in a position to burn stored fat for energy, the high heart rate of sprinting, cycling, or full-court basketball means you'll be burning the glycogen stores in your liver, and the average person only has about 50 minutes of stored energy.

Brett Fischer PT, ATC, CSCS

Brett Fischer is a licensed physical therapist, certified athletic trainer, and certified strength and conditioning specialist. He has worked with the University of Florida, the New York Jets, the Professional Golfers' Association (PGA) and Senior Tour, and the Chicago Cubs. He has served as a consultant to the San Francisco Giants and currently provides training and treatment to Major League Baseball (MLB), National Football League (NFL), National Hockey League (NHL), and National Basketball Association (NBA) athletes. Brett's expertise has led to national speaking engagements, television and radio appearances, and mention in *ESPN The Magazine*.

Brett approaches training and treatment from a total body, functional viewpoint. His professional and experienced medical staff finds and treats the source of dysfunction and pain, not just the symptoms.

Every patient/client that enters Fischer Sports Physical Therapy and Conditioning receives a thorough, functional biomechanical analysis and the appropriate medical intervention via the use of manual therapy techniques, modalities, and functional therapeutic exercises (strengthening and flexibility), as well as nutrition and diet counseling.

He recommends the following critical keys to success for athletes of all levels:

- Nutrition is paramount, whether you are talking about optimizing performance or recovery. From Brett's perspective, he works "from the outside of the body going in" and "nutrition works from the inside going out."

- Supplementation is critical, especially for professional athletes, because they don't necessarily have the time with travel to eat properly, and the demands on their bodies are so high. Brett's experience with nutrition is demonstrated by his results with two Major League Baseball (MLB) players. He worked with professional players, both of whom were under the age of twenty-five, for forty-five days and did a dietary analysis. For forty-eight hours, he tracked everything that went into their bodies—including the amount of water and the foods they consumed—and gave all the statistics to a university research center. Upon analysis, neither of the players examined met the nutritional requirements of a forty-year-old, sedentary man. This proved the importance of supplementation to the medical staff of the MLB team.

- The nutritional aspect of training is critical, because it enhances performance every single day. Brett and his staff tell athletes, "If you don't have a nutritional back-ground to stay on pace with what we're doing, then within 2-3 weeks we're going to hit a crossroads, and you're going to be sick or hurt." That's why they encourage supplementation, proper food and water intake, and proper sleep. To them, it's critical, and something they look at on a daily basis. "I believe in this stuff; that's why I do it every day," Brett explains.

- It's all about oxygenation—the more an athlete's body is oxygenized, the better the performance and recovery. They have built nitric oxide supplementation into their program, from the perspective that if they can deliver oxygen—one of the biggest things in physical therapy—more oxygen will get to the tissue and athletes will heal. That is why physical therapists do hot packs, whirlpools, and ultrasound massage. "That's the bottom line and why we recommend nitric oxide supplementation to enhance these processes," Brett explains.

So, it's vital to fuel your body for speed by consuming fiber-rich, complex carbohydrates such as whole grains and beans. These foods take longer to digest and release their energy more slowly than fast-burning, simple carbohydrates like white sugar and potatoes. Among other things, this means a steadier release of insulin to convert food into glycogen and fewer blood sugar highs and lows. Ideally, speed athletes should consume 55%-60% of their daily calories in the form of complex carbohydrates.

Listed below are some specific foods that aid in optimizing your speed:

- **Berries**—Blueberries, blackberries, and strawberries are all rich in antioxidants that can help prevent cellular damage due to the free radicals created by an intense speed workout. These compounds, known as anthocyanins, also help repair muscles after a workout, leading to stronger muscles and better performance.

- **Sweet potatoes**—Rich in Vitamin A, iron, and potassium, these colorful tubers should replace white potatoes in your diet. They are low on the glycemic index, so they don't cause insulin spikes and also enable you to digest food more steadily for more predictable energy. Sweet potatoes are also great sources of manganese, a mineral that is important for optimal cellular function.

- **Salmon and other oily fish**—Your muscles need protein to gain mass and rebuild after a tough workout, and oily fish, like salmon and tuna, are ideal lean sources of that important protein. They are also excellent sources of Omega-3 fatty acids, which reduce inflammation and can help prevent muscle soreness and injury the day after a competition.

- **Lentils**—In soups or side dishes, lentils are one of the most healthful foods you can eat—perfect for vegans or vegetarians. These tiny legumes are excellent sources of protein and contain high levels of magnesium, folic acid, and iron. Magnesium is essential to healthy cardiac function, folic acid aids in tissue regeneration, and iron is important for healthy red blood cells.

- **Healthy oils**—Sticking to a "Mediterranean" diet rich in fish and fresh vegetables is not only beneficial because it's low in fat and high in nutrients, but also because it features generous portions of healthy oils. Avocado oil, extra-virgin olive oil, and sesame oil contain plentiful levels of monounsaturated and polyunsaturated fats, which are not only good for blood sugar and blood pressure but have an anti-inflammatory effect on tissues.

It's important to remember that these are guidelines for a long-term dietary program, not for pre-race carbo-loading or eating during a competitive event. For in-event needs in particular, a whole category of gels, bars, and drinks has sprung up to provide athletes with the easily digestible, short-term energy they require. However, consuming a balanced array of nutrients as part of a regular dietary strategy has an important benefit during the rigors of intense training or competition.

As an athlete, you are probably aware that, when the body is under stress and craving quick energy during a triathlon or a soccer match, it is all too easy to reach for the nearest source of quick sugar or electrolytes. Unfortunately, these are usually not healthful foods. More often than not, they are fast foods, foods high in sugar, or packaged junk foods high in sodium—or all of the above. In consuming such foods, which promote inflammation and cause blood sugar spikes, athletes can increase their risk of poor performance and poor recovery…*unless* they have put themselves in a position to counter such effects with good, long-term dietary nutrition.

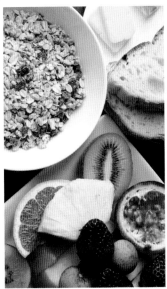

When you spend a year eating fresh fruits and vegetables, lean proteins, healthy oils, and whole grains, your body can more easily shake off the effects of a candy bar or soft drink during the course of a game. With your cells stocked with ample supplies of vital nutrients, a few unhealthy foods are far less likely to impact your performance or resilience. A sound, balanced dietary strategy thus becomes a sort of kitchen-based insurance policy for the speed-oriented athlete.

Featured Athlete: Chris McCormack, 2010 Ironman™ World Champion

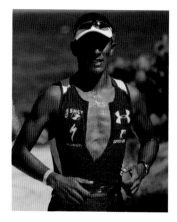

Probably the greatest triathlete in the history of the sport, Chris "Macca" McCormack may be best known for endurance, not speed. But now that he is competing against athletes half his age to make the 2012 Olympics in short-course triathlon, speed is a far more critical element of his game. We interviewed him by email to learn his secrets.

What is your daily workout routine?

I spend about six hours per day on average training. My routine varies from day to day but usually involves a minimum of two disciplines: swim-bike, bike-run, or swim-run. Intensity and volume depend upon my training plan, but multi-sport athletes tend to train a lot. I sleep about eight hours per night, and my training usually starts early so as to ensure I have some break in the middle of the day between sessions. On heavy days I can be working out for up to ten hours.

What is your typical daily diet?

I eat a very balanced diet. I am not a difficult person when it comes to eating. For triathletes, the focus is on getting enough calories to sustain the amount of work we are doing, while keeping our weight in check. I eat very healthily and am aware of what I am eating. I honestly think this is the best thing. I try to ensure that at least 80%-90% of the time I am eating well. I attach no guilt to my eating. I think guilt is a much bigger issue than what you actually eat.

Do you use dietary supplements? If so, which ones?

I really only use a single dietary supplement: a colostrum-based product out of Germany. Pre-race, I will use a Coenzyme Q10 load of about 5000 mg per day for about five days out. Magnesium and potassium help with hydration for my races.

What foods do you eat and what supplements do you take to promote recovery, allowing you to train with greater intensity while preventing injury?

I ensure that post-workout I rehydrate with a carbohydrate solution with electrolytes. This helps restore my lost glycogen. After big sessions I do take in a protein shake—a whey protein with a small portion of soy protein—but my main focus is ensuring that I eat well.

How do you maintain your optimal performance level with the travel demands of your sport?

Travel is the most difficult thing on a racer. It is tough, but you have to be able to adapt to your surroundings well and release your rigid mindset. By being flexible in your training routine and understanding that sticking to a strict program on the road is a recipe for disaster, you can adapt quickly. I have training bases around the world; this makes intercontinental travel easy. When I am racing in Europe for prolonged times, I usually train out of Wiesbaden, Germany. This really feels like a home away from home, so my transition into a training environment is easy. In the U.S., Los Angeles is my home. Having familiar places to go to allows you to get back into a routine very quickly.

What aspects of your fitness and nutrition program do you consider most important for getting the results you want (e.g., core training for preventing injury, etc.)?

Flexibility in your program. I think rigidity in anything is a recipe for disaster. You need to ensure that you are doing the key sessions or eating the correct foods, but attaching guilt to anything is just prehistoric thinking, in my opinion. Your body and fitness are holistic, and trying to single out individual things or sessions is impossible.

The key to prolonged success is making a constant assessment of your strengths and weaknesses and then making sure you address these in the next phase of your training. I don't believe in the fitness principle of *periodization*.

I think the human body responds better to consistency of work, with changed and different stresses, to achieve a platform of strength and health. I think this is the key to remaining injury-free. Have consistency across everything and trust in your body's rhythms. If you're tired, rest. Athletes fear rest too much. If you're injured, have it treated and don't rush back to working out because of fear. Have faith in your overall fitness program and your ability as an athlete to endure. Not enough focus is given to an athlete's frame of mind in winning events.

From a nutritional and exercise perspective, what would you recommend to the young athlete or weekend warrior who wants to take his or her performance to the next level?

I encourage people to be aware of what they eat on both a balanced nutrient level and a volume level. I don't believe in specific diets, but I do believe that eating well is imperative. When I say well, this means both the amount you consume and the quality of the food you consume. Keeping the refined foods to a minimum is something I am very focused on. Staying as close to fresh as possible is always good, and organic is great. Understanding your perfect performance weight is a foundation to work from, too. You should know your perfect race weight. Making sure that your body is fueled well is a great starting point for any weekend warrior.

On an exercise level, a focus on consistency in aerobic exercise is a prerequisite to success. Consistency is key, so that you can hold a basic level of fitness at all times. You can fit a training program and structure around this, but having a base fitness level to start from, grown out of consistent physical activity, allows you to build the harder sessions around your weaknesses and gives you a stronger foundation.

Focus on strength over speed as a weekend warrior. For younger athletes, nailing the technique and biomechanics of the triathlon sports is the most important thing. Then add speed to the equation, followed by strength. Strength will come with age and consistency. The key is to make sure that young athletes develop good habits, initiate their speed, and build strength and endurance with time. The key word, across the board, is *consistency*.

What is your greatest sports moment?

Winning the ITU Triathlon World Championships (my first world title) as a 23-year-old boy. It was a lifelong goal, and it ranked me as the best athlete in the world for my sport. It was the first time I had tasted this, and to fulfill a dream like that is amazing. I went on to win world titles at Ironman™, but this first world title is my most treasured.

What are the top three things you would recommend to a recreationally elite athlete to improve performance as he or she ages?

1. Range of Motion—You lose flexibility as you age, so making sure you address this as you train is crucial. The more you can maintain your range of motion, the longer you can perform. Don't go crazy with it, but addressing it on a daily basis for a small period of time is great.

2. Strength—Maintaining your strength is essential. Even doing some time in the gym to generate the hormonal response of power work is good. Strength and power work are easier to do and will give you a lot of benefits as you age.

3. Rest—You can't do the volume of work you did when you were younger. You require a little more time between tougher sessions, and recovery becomes a much more important piece of the puzzle. Rest needs to become a bigger friend as you age. For example, if you have always worked off a seven-day training cycle, as you age, you may do the same volume and intensity of work over eight or nine days.

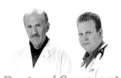

Doctors' Comments

Chris McCormack is an incredible athlete, both in terms of his speed and endurance on land and in the water. His many hours of weekly exercise on the bike, in the pool, and on the road give him sky-high levels of NO, which enables him to put forth bursts of speed when necessary. However, like many triathletes, this level of activity also produces high levels of free radicals in his tissues. The antioxidants in his healthful diet help prevent cellular damage, which is one reason he has rarely been injured. Athletes who aspire to the same combination of speed, endurance, and durability would do well to supplement with NO and antioxidants to both enable better anaerobic performance and prevent oxidative damage.

Power Nutrients for Speed

Because intense speed training and competition so readily deplete the body of key nutrients, athletes who desire peak performance should not limit their nutritional intake to dietary sources alone. Despite the news that supplement use is currently falling among athletes, we would like to see this trend reversed. As more and more athletes become aware of the importance of augmenting dietary nutrients with unadulterated nutrients in supplement form, we believe this will occur.

There are several Power Nutrients that have been shown to be beneficial for the sprinter, runner, or other type of athlete seeking to increase speed. They are:

- **Antioxidants**—As part of natural mitochondrial respiration, the process by which chemical reactions produce fuel for our cells, various types of free radicals form in the tissues. Exercise amplifies this effect while depleting the body's supplies of antioxidants. Antioxidants are the body's main defense against the cell-damaging properties of these molecules, which is why the foundation of antioxidant intake must be a widely varied diet rich in colorful fruits and vegetables.

  With more than 5,000 identified antioxidants, it would be impossible to get a sufficient variety through supplementation alone. However, supplements play a vital protective role by adding powerful antioxidants such as alpha lipoic acid and epigallocatechin gallate (EGCG) from green tea in high concentrations. Supplements also backstop dietary consumption by ensuring adequate intake of antioxidants in case of dietary insufficiency due to travel or other demands.

- **Creatine**—Creatine phosphate is one of the primary fuels for the kind of short-term muscle use that occurs during sprints, speed skating, and other intense, speed-based sporting activities. Unfortunately, natural creatine levels in the body decline with age, leaving athletes with less quick-release energy for short-burst, high-intensity workouts or competitions. Added to the natural decline in fast-twitch muscle fiber and stride length that also come with the passage of time, it's easy to see why speed-based athletes tend to lose their ability to remain competitive at high levels sooner than endurance athletes do.

Interestingly, it appears that rigorous speed and power training can actually reverse some of this creatine phosphate decline. Research has shown that, by doing six weeks of cycle training, a group of athletes ranging from ages of sixty-one to eighty increased their creatine phosphate levels to those of younger adults. This suggests that regular, intense speed training may be part of the remedy for age-related creatine decline.

However, numerous studies have shown that creatine supplementation increases muscle power and sustained power through anaerobic repetition. In one important study, Schedel et al. examined the results of four consecutive sprints by seven sprinters after one week of either creatine supplementation or a placebo. The runners who took the creatine supplement increased their running speed by 1.4% and their stride frequency or turnover by 1.5% over the placebo runners. The researchers concluded that creatine supplementation could shorten muscular relaxation time, leading to faster contractions and better sprint times.

- **Omega-3 fatty acids**—Essential fatty acids are powerful anti-inflammatory agents, and therein lies their value for the speed-based athlete. While there is some research that suggests that polyunsaturated fatty acids, such as those found in sunflower oil (the type of oil used in the study), may increase maximum running speed in Olympic sprinters, no mechanism for that increase has been validated yet. We prefer to focus on the heavily supported fact of Omega-3 fatty acids for preventing inflammatory damage to tissues.

  Quite simply, speed workouts damage muscles, resulting in inflammation and soreness. By minimizing this tissue inflammation, a diet rich in Omega-3 fatty acids can both reduce post-workout pain (allowing more intense, more frequent workouts) and reduce the risk of injury. Consumption of Omega-3 fatty acids has also been shown to speed up the body's basal metabolic rate, aiding in fat loss and the maintenance of lean body mass—an obvious competitive advantage for runners.

- **L-arginine**—The impact of arginine on running speed and performance is really a matter of simple math. When your muscles are working anaerobically (without oxygen), one unit of glucose produces two units of energy with lactic acid as the by-product. Lactic acid slows muscle contractions and creates fatigue. When your muscles are working aerobically (with oxygen), one glucose unit creates 36 units of energy with CO_2 and water as the by-products. Since lactic acid buildup can negatively impact performance, athletes are best served by training and nutritional efforts that maximize blood flow, thereby delivering more oxygen and nutrients to the muscles. This allows athletes to work at a high aerobic capacity for longer periods and engage in high-intensity exercise or "surges" (as in sprint races) with less lactic acid buildup.

  As we have already seen, supplementation with arginine optimizes the ability of the endothelium, the lining of the blood vessels, to produce nitric oxide, or NO, the powerful gas that relaxes and expands vessel walls to allow for greater circulatory volume. Consuming sufficient arginine through supplements improves NO production and blood flow, allowing the muscles, tissues, and organs used during all phases of competitive running to perform more efficiently and recover more quickly.

- **Protein**—The great majority of the protein needed for speed workouts and competition will, of course, be consumed via an athlete's normal diet. However, supplementation addresses the need for *rapid* protein delivery at a higher rate of absorption. Consumption of supplements of whey protein can address these needs.

Power Nutrients for Speed

- Antioxidants, including CoQ10
- Creatine
- EFAs
- L-arginine
- Protein

Chapter Six
Nutrition and Strength

Muscular strength is essential to virtually all sporting pursuits, from team sports such as football and baseball, to sports that emphasize explosiveness such as basketball, track, field, and martial arts. Even endurance sports like a triathlon have a strength component, because strength in athletes is simply the controlled application of mechanical force to a resistant surface or object. In running, it's the ground. In swimming, it's the water. In baseball, it's the ball. In boxing, it's your opponent's face.

Strength (or power) also comes into play in training. Much of the training regimen for any athlete will be resistance training: the lifting of weight to cause muscle contractions. These can include weight lifting (bench-presses, squats), body weight exercises (pushups, pull-ups), and core exercises (crunches, yoga poses). Over time, such action damages muscle fibers, and the recovery from that damage through rest, hydration, and nutrition leads to muscle growth, increased metabolism, greater strength, and increased lean body mass.

Greater muscle strength also reduces the risk of injury as muscles are better able to support the joints and skeletal system and more resistant to exercise-induced trauma. According to the Mayo Clinic, strength training also improves muscle tone and coordination and reduces the decline in muscle mass that usually accompanies age.

Strength and Sports

Because the application of muscular force is anaerobic, strength-related exercise causes the buildup of lactic acid in the muscles. Depending on its duration, intense exercise requiring power and explosiveness—ski jumping, volleyball, powerlifting—taps into one of two anaerobic energy systems, neither of which rely on oxygen as a catalyst for the chemical reaction that produces energy. As the muscles are pushed to failure (pain or the inability to further contract without rest), lactic acid accumulates in the tissues. Beyond a certain threshold (the *lactate threshold*) lactic acid begins to cause fatigue, thereby negatively impacting performance.

This may not have a noticeable effect on casual exercisers, who either do not engage in anaerobic exercise intense enough to cause lactic acid buildup at sufficient levels or engage primarily in aerobic exercise, which does not cause lactate accumulation. However, the rigorous workouts and competitive performance of athletes, pro or amateur, makes the lactate threshold relevant.

Because of this biological reality, training and nutrition that improves the ability of muscles to contract powerfully for longer periods, before failure, is highly beneficial to athletes in almost any sport, as most sports require strength in some manner. Intense physical training has been shown to optimize the anaerobic system, which is why endurance athletes focus obsessively on workouts that raise their lactate thresholds. But even sports that do not appear to be strength-based can benefit from exercise and dietary solutions that promote strength:

- **Golf**—Despite its perception as a non-athlete's sport, golfing at high levels requires tremendous rotational power through the core, torso, and shoulders in order to generate the force necessary to hit a golf ball in excess of 300 yards. While muscle failure may not come into play given the game's pace, muscular endurance comes into play in promoting precision and accuracy over 18 holes.

- **Swimming**—Strength translates into propulsion in swimming, where the force a swimmer is able to exert against the resistance of the water determines how fast he or she is able to go. Power through the chest, shoulders, arms, and upper back is critical at the higher levels of the sport.

- **Skiing**—We often associate skiing with agility and endurance, but great lower body and core strength is needed for professionals or elite amateurs to carve turns in deep powder or over long slalom or mogul courses in competition.

- **Triathlon**—The ultimate endurance sport, triathlon nevertheless has numerous instances where muscle strength can make the difference between winning and losing, particularly in the swimming and biking stages. Swimming demands the power referenced above, while passing and climbing in cycling require exceptional lower body power.

Whether it's upper body power, core strength, or lower body explosiveness, muscular strength is critical to peak performance in most sports, making a nutritional strategy that optimizes strength and muscle recovery a necessary part of any athlete's program.

NO and Strength

Nitric oxide plays a central role in the development and display of athletic strength. First of all, strength is gained through muscle development, which in turn, occurs when muscles are damaged at the microscopic level through training and then recovery. By promoting oxygen and nutrient delivery, NO helps muscle damage heal more quickly so that new muscle can form. The molecule also enhances circulation to training muscles so athletes can lift more and lift longer, resulting in greater gains.

During sports activity, NO regulates the function of mitochondria, the energy generators for each cell, enabling each cell to utilize blood glucose and stored glycogen energy at top efficiency, extracting the most possible work from each calorie. Finally, NO helps to clear lactic acid from tissues. As you know, lactic acid buildup occurs when the anaerobic energy system is engaged, and too much lactic acid causes fatigue and muscle failure. By delaying this buildup, NO enables athletes to exert strength both longer and at greater intensity levels.

Paired with protective antioxidants, NO allows bodybuilders, cyclists, football players, and other strength-based athletes to train more, train harder, and put out more strength on the field or track.

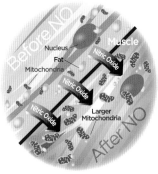

Nitric Oxide Supports Muscle Energy

Nitric Oxide supports muscle energy by enhancing mitochondrial activity.

Eating for Strength

The goals of athletes seeking to build strength are typically twofold: to build muscle while keeping body weight low. The more you weigh, the more energy it takes to propel that weight through the motions of your sport. And, since fat does not exert force, it follows that reducing body fat must be a dietary goal alongside developing muscle.

For most athletes, this means escaping the three meals per day mindset. Instead, most fitness trainers and conditioning coaches recommend eating between five and eight meals per day, based on your calorie needs. The formula you use to calculate the calories you require per day will depend on a number of variables: your body type, metabolism, sport, training intensity, and goals. For example, a man trying to add 20 pounds of lean muscle will need to consume more calories each day than a woman trying to lose body fat.

The trick here is balance: eat enough quality calories throughout the day to keep your metabolism running at a high level while not overeating and storing body fat. Eating consistent, small meals helps burn more fat in the long run, because 70% of the calories you burn daily are used to simply operate your body in what's called the *thermic effect of food.*

The types of food to eat is a simpler matter. First of all, muscle and strength-building are about protein. Protein builds, maintains, and repairs muscle tissue and also serves as a secondary energy source. To repair the damage caused by rigorous exercise and add lean body mass, you need to consume as many grams per day of quality protein as your desired body weight in pounds. So, if your goal is a lean body weight of 185 pounds, you should be consuming 185 grams of protein daily, spread out among five to eight meals, and eaten every two to three hours.

Here are some ideal strength building foods:

- **Lean meat**—Poultry, such as chicken and turkey, can provide up to 30 grams of protein per serving with a low saturated fat content. Grass-fed beef is another excellent lean protein source, because it typically contains high levels of Omega-3 fatty acids as well as abundant protein. Be sure to grill or bake your meat, rather than fry it, to reduce calories.

- **Fish**—Salmon, anchovies, tuna, sardines, cod, tilapia, and halibut are some of the best options for athletes after their daily protein fix. Many types of fish such as salmon and mackerel, also deliver high levels of Omega-3 fatty acids, whose anti-inflammatory properties can alleviate joint pain and fatigue while speeding up metabolism and helping to burn fat. Fish also tends to be lower in calories than meats such as beef or pork.

- **Egg whites**—In general, concern about the high cholesterol content of egg yolks is misplaced, because dietary cholesterol has not been linked to high levels of serum cholesterol in the blood. However, if you are reluctant to consume the whole egg, egg whites provide a nearly pure protein source with no fat and all nine essential amino acids. A typical egg white contains about four to five grams of protein. You can also buy pasteurized egg whites in cartons at the grocery store, an option that's easier and faster for busy athletes after their morning protein.

- **Complex Carbohydrates**—Food by itself does not build muscle. Workouts build muscle, and your body relies on stored glycogen for fuel during demanding resistance workouts. Eat sufficient complex carbohydrates at each meal. These carbohydrates digest slowly and release their energy gradually, providing long-term fuel to muscles during difficult exercise. Eating carbohydrates after a workout, along with protein, also helps your body better absorb the protein and store energy. Examples of quality complex carbohydrates include brown rice, sweet potatoes, quinoa, oatmeal, and fiber-rich vegetables like broccoli.

- **Nuts**—Nuts are an ideal protein source for athletes who don't eat meat. Because they are dense in calories, athletes trying to control body weight should eat them in moderation; nonetheless, nuts contain substantial protein as well as high levels of healthy fats that reduce inflammation and improve cardiovascular health. University of Arizona research suggests almonds or walnuts are the best choices for athletes trying to build muscle mass, though most nuts are powerhouses of important minerals and fiber.

In general, if you are trying to develop greater strength and power, eat breakfast each day: an egg white omelet, a protein shake, or oatmeal and raw berries. A healthy breakfast revs up your metabolism while fueling exercise later in the day. Also, avoid many of the bars and shakes on the market; some are extremely high in calories and sugar. Instead, try to make 90% of your diet whole foods: fresh fruits and vegetables, raw juices, whole grains, low-fat dairy, nuts, seeds, legumes, and some lean meat. Finally, drink enough water—at least 8-12 8oz. glasses daily. Water helps your kidneys excrete the excess protein that your body does not convert into muscle, helps you feel full, and prevents dehydration, which can harm performance.

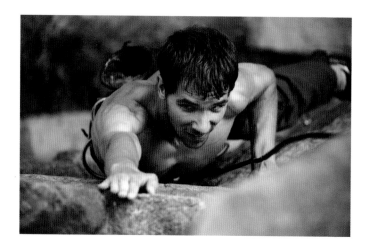

Featured Athlete: Lauren Megale Jones, Top-Ranked NCAA Tennis Player

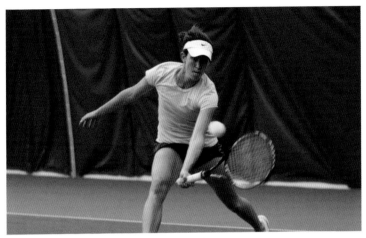

Lauren Megale Jones has excelled at collegiate tennis at both Arizona State University and later, at Boise State University, dominating in Western Athletic Conference competition and ranking as high as 14th in the nation among eighteen-year-olds. As she begins her professional career, she shares her training secrets for a sport that requires speed, agility, endurance, and, above all, strength.

What is your daily workout routine?

It varies from day to day, and it changes if I have a tournament coming up. However, there is a five-hour time period spent training daily. I do weights and conditioning for one and a half hours—weights three days a week and conditioning every day. I spend three to three and a half hours on the court a day, one-and-a-half in the morning and two in the afternoon. At the end, there is a thirty-minute stretch, but I stretch before and after every workout.

What is your typical daily diet?

No fast food whatsoever. No soda. I have a sweet tooth, so cutting out goodies is hard for me to do. I always eat a well-balanced breakfast: an English muffin with peanut butter, scrambled eggs, milk, and daily vitamins. I have a very fast metabolism, so I eat before lunch with a snack of some sort (bar, nuts, or a smoothie). Lunch is random. I do not eat a lot for lunch; a typical day includes a sandwich, soup, and a lot of water. Dinner lately has been steak, vegetables, and potatoes. I also enjoy chicken Parmesan and zucchini. Before a tournament, I eat pasta with chicken mixed in, and drink a lot of water.

Do you use dietary supplements? If so, which ones?

I use a carbohydrate sports drink during competition, and I drink a meal replacement drink because my metabolism burns calories quickly; it is hard to stay energized in a three-hour tennis match without proper fuel. I also take gel during competition, but no other dietary supplements.

What foods do you eat and what supplements do you take to promote recovery, allowing you to train with greater intensity while preventing injury?

I love to drink chocolate milk or a protein drink after a hard lift. I like to drink a carbohydrate drink before and after competition because it helps my muscles to prepare and recover after a long day on the courts. I will take glucosamine supplements if my muscles are really torn up, but it's not something I take daily. I also like to eat pineapple for recovery.

How do you maintain your optimal performance level with the travel demands of your sport?

We travel a lot, so I make sure I get into a rhythm. I buy the same groceries no matter what city we are in, and I go to the same restaurants so that I am familiar with the food I am eating. As far as international competition, I bring my essentials with me, because the chances of a foreign country having those items may be slim. I also maintain a rhythm by going to bed at the same time, practicing at the exact times I will be playing my match, and listening to the same music. Habit is huge.

What aspects of your fitness and nutrition program do you consider most important for getting the results you want (e.g., core training for preventing injury, etc.)?

Fitness: I always need to make sure that I am doing no more than three miles running straight ahead. I do a lot of change of direction drills. The legs and core are a huge part of a tennis player's build, so it is important to make sure to build a strong base with your legs and a strong core. Shoulder health is also very important, and this has to do with band work and stretching.

Nutrition: Eat a lot, all the time. I burn too much, too fast, not to be eating. Healthy eating is essential to proper energy levels—water, fruit, protein, and a controlled amount of carbohydrates.

From a nutritional and exercise perspective, what would you recommend to the young athlete or weekend warrior who wants to take his or her performance to the next level?

Start creating good habits right away, because they will stay with you for the rest of your life. Wake up early and do training that no one else wants to do. Eat healthily, and get sleep!

What is your greatest sports moment?

I have had a lot of special moments as a tennis player, but one that comes to mind is when I won my first national championship in Texas. I played really tough the whole week under hot weather conditions and against difficult opponents, and I stayed focused mentally. I beat tough players right before my freshman year of college. It was a great motivator for the college tennis I was about to experience.

What are the top three things you would recommend to a recreationally elite athlete to improve performance as he or she ages?

Train smart. More hours doesn't mean you are getting better. Quality over quantity training takes an athlete a long way. Have fun while you are training. If you are not having fun, then you are not going to get the most out of the sport. Compete. The only way to get better is to compete. Play competitive games in everything, not just the sport you compete in. This will make you a better competitor for your primary sport, and it will give you opportunities to get put in situations that could help you in a crucial moment in the future.

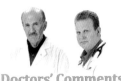

Doctors' Comments

Lauren's sport, tennis, is one of the most demanding on the body. On demand, she must be able to exhibit speed, strength, flexibility, quickness, and precision—and in long matches, exceptional endurance. She sounds like she could stand to consume more calories, but NO supplementation would also help her body make better use of the calories she takes in. As she heads for the ranks of pro tennis, Power Nutrients could be a difference maker. For tennis players of a more ordinary level, NO supplementation can improve power, speed, and endurance.

Power Nutrients for Strength

The ideal Power Nutrients contributing to strength and muscle power are those that either promote muscle growth or optimize the metabolic pathways that deliver fuel and oxygen to working muscles:

- **Citrulline**—Many athletes (especially bodybuilders) train while supplementing with citrulline malate, which can be consumed in watermelon and apples, but is more plentiful via dietary supplements. Citrulline is a precursor to arginine, which, as we have seen, increases production of nitric oxide (NO) in the endothelium. NO, in turn, relaxes blood vessels, increasing nutrient and oxygen uptake by tissues. Citrulline also exerts a protective effect on arginine by deactivating arginase, an enzyme that destroys arginine molecules. This leaves more arginine available to exert its beneficial effects on the body.

  Citrulline has also been shown to boost levels of ATP (*adenosine triphosphate*), the chemical key to cellular energy. This can result in greater muscle endurance, more reps, and better muscle development. Citrulline also reduces lactic acid buildup, which helps stave off fatigue and allows athletes to train or compete longer.

- **Creatine**—Clinical studies suggest that creatine supplementation increases lean muscle mass as well as athletic performance, though it does not appear to assist with endurance-based performance like distance running. Laboratory studies indicate that creatine supplements improve strength and the development of lean muscle mass during high-intensity, short duration exercises like weightlifting.

  Typically taken in powder form, and usually mixed with fruit juice, creatine appears to be most beneficial for strength-oriented athletes in the weight room, where it allows for more rigorous, longer training sessions that build more powerful musculature. Other proven benefits of creatine include longer anaerobic respiration of muscle cells, more resistance repetitions, faster sprint times, higher lean body mass, and quicker recovery.

- **Protein**—Apart from plentiful amounts of protein in the diet, athletes can benefit from protein supplementation consumed at the right times, typically just following a workout. One of the most common supplements is whey isolate in powder form, which is about 90% protein, mixed with fruit juice or added into a shake with other ingredients. Taken after a workout, the extra protein is readily absorbed by the damaged muscles and aids in recovery and the growth of new muscle tissue. Protein supplements can also be taken before a workout for additional energy.

Protein has numerous functions in the body in addition to muscle building. It helps maintain proper hormone levels, balances blood acidity, catalyzes important chemical reactions, boosts the immune system, preserves muscle tissue, maintains levels of essential amino acids, and regulates fluid balance. Consuming sufficient protein not only ensures that these vital functions continue, but protein is also highly thermogenic, meaning that its digestion burns more calories than the digestion of carbohydrates or fats. So, eating sufficient protein in all forms can increase base metabolism and help create more lean body mass in the long term.

- **BCAA**—Consuming branched-chain amino acids during strength training appears to increase muscle strength as well as lean body mass, the twin goals of most athletes. A 2009, randomized, double-blind study put 36 men experienced in weight training through an eight-week resistance training program involving all major muscle groups. During the program, some of the men were given BCAA, while some were given whey protein and others carbohydrates. At the conclusion of the study, the men who had received BCAA had gained significantly more lean body mass, lost more body fat, and gained significantly more strength on the bench press and squat than the men who had received protein or carbohydrate supplements.

- **Glutamine**—As discussed in Section 1, glutamine has numerous benefits in the areas of muscle development, weight loss, development of lean body mass, and overall strength training results. Glutamine is abundant in the body, but it is also easily depleted through exercise. According to research by Roth, intense exercise can deplete glutamine by 40%-50%. This is dangerous because, not only do the muscles use glutamine as a major component of the post-workout rebuilding process, but the immune system also relies on the amino acid. So, overtraining, leading to a glutamine deficiency, can cause an immune system deficiency as well as muscle wasting.

For athletes, glutamine is an important supplement because it promotes glycogen formation and protein synthesis, prevents the consumption of muscle tissue for energy, and boosts levels of growth hormones. It is clear that for athletes training rigorously for maximum strength while preventing injury, illness, and muscle damage, those are desirable benefits.

Power Nutrients for Strength

- L-citrulline
- Creatine
- Protein
- BCAA (Branched-Chain Amino Acid)
- L-glutamine

Chapter Seven
Nutrition and Endurance

Triathletes. Marathoners. Boxers. Distance swimmers. Cyclists. All of these are athletes for whom endurance is central to their athletic endeavors. Endurance is simply the ability to sustain a consistent level of exertion for a long period of time.

There are four types of endurance: aerobic, anaerobic, speed, and strength. All involve producing ATP as fuel from glucose in the bloodstream and glycogen stored in the muscles. But each has a different mechanism and places different demands on the body:

- **Aerobic** endurance exercise is done at a level at which the body relies on fuel intake and oxygen, creating very little waste. The longer aerobic work continues, the more it relies purely on the aerobic systems and less on the anaerobic for energy. Aerobic endurance is built using long-term distance exercise such as running and cycling, which improves the body's maximum oxygen uptake, known as VO2Max, and interval training, which optimizes the heart's ability to pump blood.

  Aerobic endurance exercises typically involve lower-intensity exertion that can last for long periods, while maintaining the heart rate at no more than about 65% of maximum, to avoid engaging the anaerobic system and creating fatigue-producing waste products. While the heart rates of marathon runners and other endurance athletes can and do exceed 150 beats per minute during competition, they rarely reach the high rates of athletes whose sports are based on explosive "surges" of short-term strength or speed.

Aerobic endurance typically comes into play in distance sports such as triathlon, running, cycling, cross-country skiing, sculling, and swimming.

- **Anaerobic** endurance work occurs when the body is working at a high enough intensity that systems must use the fuel stored in muscles as glycogen, thereby reaching the anaerobic or lactate threshold. This quickly results in oxygen debt and lactic acid accumulation, which leads to muscle fatigue and eventual failure.

  The duration of anaerobic endurance work is very short, as muscle tissues typically contain little more than four seconds of stored energy at maximum effort. Even long-term anaerobic endurance exercise will last for no more than one to two minutes (rowing races, 400-meter sprints, wrestling) and will also engage the aerobic energy system.

  Athletes needing to build their anaerobic endurance will do so typically with high-intensity intervals of resistance-based training, combined with short recovery periods.

  Anaerobic endurance is commonly relied on by athletes in such sports as basketball, soccer, baseball, and lacrosse, where long periods of moderate aerobic work can give way to short bursts of intense speed and power.

- **Speed** endurance basically reflects the ability of muscles to contract more rapidly, such as in 800-meter races and other long sprints. Speed endurance is highly anaerobic, given that training to increase contraction speed involves heavy repetition at high intensity, typically multiple intervals at 80% of maximum heart rate and higher.

  Speed endurance comes into play in sports that require sustained exertion of speed for more than sprint duration, such as track and field and speed skating.

- **Strength** endurance is about developing the ability to sustain the contraction force of the muscles over time. This is vital for all athletes, as even marathoners and ultra-distance runners have a periodic need for "surges" of power during races. Strength endurance develops via disciplines such as weight training and circuit training. Strength endurance is relevant for all sports, as it centers on the ability to repeat powerful muscle contractions for as long as possible before failure, something vital in running, jumping, climbing, cycling, and the like.

What we usually think of as endurance exercise—running on a treadmill, long-distance kayaking, etc.—is actually built on aerobic endurance. This activity uses the slow-twitch muscles: blood-rich tissues that are highly aerobic and are fueled using ample supplies of oxygen. Slow-twitch muscles are more efficient at using oxygen to produce fuel than the fast-twitch muscles used in sprinting and other explosive exercises. They fire more slowly and contract less violently than fast-twitch muscles, so they fatigue less easily.

Because of this, typical endurance activity is at a steady pace and is prepared for by long, slow distance training punctuated with intervals of high-intensity training. This improves cardiovascular fitness and capacity while fostering the growth of new blood vessels that better transport oxygen and nutrients to the cells.

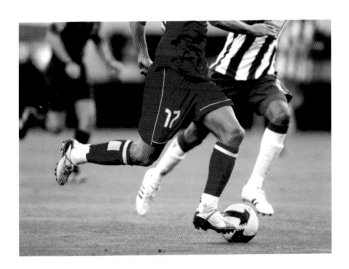

Featured Athlete: Michelle Macy, Marathon Swimmer

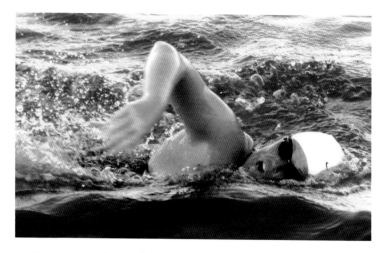

Having swum the English Channel and the Strait of Gibraltar and participated as part of a relay team in the five-day, five-Ironman™, five-island challenge known as EPIC5, Michelle Macy has become one of the world's elite cold-water distance swimmers. She shares her training and dietary secrets:

What is your daily workout routine?

- Monday and Wednesday: 5:15a.m.-6:45a.m., swim practice with "US Marathon Swimmers (USMS)" team, then a half to one and a half hour "prehab" program to maintain shoulder and overall body health.
- Tuesday and Thursday: 6:00a.m.-7:00a.m. Pilates class, 7:00a.m.-8:00a.m functional training class.
- Friday: Long pool or open water workout. The time, intensity, and focus of this workout depends on the upcoming marathon swim on the schedule. This is followed by the half to one and a half hour prehab program.
- Saturday: Long pool or open water workout. The time, intensity, and focus of this workout depend on the upcoming marathon swim on the schedule.
- Sunday: Recovery day, or, as I like to call it, catch up on everything else day, as training and a full-time job leave little time during the week to do other necessary tasks.

What is your typical daily diet?
- Pre-workout: I usually eat a nutritional bar and drink water.
- Post- workout: I try to eat a good, nutritional breakfast: oatmeal with dried fruit and cinnamon, or a bagel with ham and/or turkey. I load up on water as well.
- 10:00a.m.-11:00a.m.: I eat a small snack. I try to make it nutritious, (e.g., a piece of fruit and some nuts).
- 11:30a.m.-1:00p.m.: Lunch. I pick this up from my work cafeteria. I look at nutrition content and work hard to ensure a balance of protein, veggies, and carbohydrates.
- 3:00p.m.: I eat a small snack.
- 5:30p.m.-7:00p.m.: Dinner. This is highly variable on content and whether homemade or takeout.

Do you use dietary supplements? If so, which ones?

Liquid calcium magnesium, a probiotic drink, and fish oil.

What foods do you eat and what supplements do you take to promote recovery, allowing you to train with greater intensity while preventing injury?

I used to do a lot more recovery drinks and such, prior to finding out that I had a few food sensitivity issues mainly related to dairy. Now, I try my best to eat normal foods soon after a workout to aid in recovery. I've also greatly increased my water intake, which has really helped my overall performance and recovery.

How do you maintain your optimal performance level with the travel demands of your sport?

I really try to maintain a similar sleep and nutrition pattern as at home. Additionally, I work to increase fluid intake to alleviate any dehydration that may occur during travel.

What aspects of your fitness and nutrition program do you consider most important for getting the results you want (e.g., core training for preventing injury, etc.)?

Most important are my swim training, injury prevention training, and recovery time. It is hard to select one aspect of my training that is the most important as I believe that the combination of all the training is crucial to my success. If one component slips, then I won't perform at the optimal level and get the results that I strive for.

From a nutritional and exercise perspective, what would you recommend to the young athlete or weekend warrior who wants to take his or her performance to the next level?

First and foremost, set a goal. From there, seek out professionals to help you achieve that goal in a healthy manner.

What is your greatest sports moment?

It's hard to narrow it down to one. However, there is one moment that I remember that turned me into a cold-water marathon swimmer: my first English Channel swim in 2007. I wasn't sure if I could actually accomplish the goal. As I was swimming along, I had one of my best friends and my parents on the boat, crewing and cheering me on. We got about a mile from France, and I had been swimming really hard, because I was afraid that I was going to miss the tide and end up swimming in place for six hours.

I looked up at my crew and said, "Did I get through?" They looked at me and said, "You're golden." It was at that moment that I knew I was going to be a true Channel swimmer. With tears and laughter and lots of love and support, I ran up onto the beach in France.

What are the top three things you would recommend to a recreationally elite athlete to improve performance as he or she ages?

1. Find a really good athletic trainer and or physical therapist who can help "pre" habilitate your body and keep it from those breakdown moments and, ultimately, avoid rehabilitation.

2. Join a group or team that will help support your goals and keep you motivated.

3. Set a goal above what you think is possible, and then set the plan to get there. So much fun will be had in the journey towards your goal.

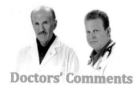

Doctors' Comments

Michelle faces different demands than athletes whose main concern is safely bleeding off excess body heat. Since she is submerged in water, heat is less of a concern than hypothermia. So, her body must be able to produce excess energy to keep vital organs and tissues warm during multi-hour swims. She does consume some Power Nutrients, but it is likely that her swimming keeps her NO levels extremely high, so supplementation would probably serve as a means to further performance. For non-elite swimmers, however, it could be a great asset. By optimizing circulation to the extremities and vital organs, NO helps the body maintain a consistent core temperature, while delivering nutrients to maintain a high activity level. Pool swimmers and open water swimmers alike would benefit from increasing their own NO stores to the level of this elite athlete.

NO and Endurance

Endurance sports are about consistency—of heart rate, respiration, and calorie consumption and replenishment—and blood flow through the vascular tree. NO signals the six billion endothelial cells in the circulatory system to relax and expand the vessel walls, lowering blood pressure and evening out flow throughout the body's systems. In this way, NO promotes consistent supply of nutrients and oxygen, as well as allows the blood to recirculate to the skin, cooling the body.

Research has shown that NO supplementation also reduces the "oxygen cost" of endurance exercise—the amount of oxygen needed to sustain the cellular reactions that power the body. Lower oxygen requirements for the same level of performance may mean that athletes whose bodies transport and utilize oxygen with greater effectiveness have a performance edge in endurance sports.

NO also reduces platelet aggregation, the condition in which platelets in the blood adhere, often the beginnings of a blood clot. As endurance athletes can be vulnerable to blood clots and deep vein thrombosis, having sufficient NO levels is important for preventing these potentially dangerous conditions.

Diet and Endurance

A diet for endurance should center on complex carbohydrates, your body's major fuel source. Ideally, at least 50% of an endurance athlete's diet should consist of complex, slow-digesting carbohydrates, such as brown rice, whole grains, oatmeal, vegetables, and legumes. A balanced endurance diet should also include sufficient lean protein to repair muscles damaged by long runs or cycling workouts, along with the healthy fats needed for cardiovascular health and preventing inflammation, leading to quicker recovery. Still, a diet high in carbohydrates will store more glycogen in muscles than any other regimen, enabling athletes to perform at higher levels on race day.

This sort of food intake is what endurance athletes should strive for. Endurance foods include:

- **Chia seeds**—Made famous in the book, *Born to Run*, chia seeds are known as the ultimate running food. They can be eaten pre-workout for easy-to-digest energy or during a workout because they are easy to transport and don't cause stomach upset. They're also packed with beneficial nutrients. Chia seeds contain high levels of antioxidants, a great deal of protein and dietary fiber, and minerals, including calcium, magnesium, and zinc. They are also gluten-free.

- **Green, leafy vegetables**—From spinach to kale to bok choy, leafy greens are perhaps the healthiest foods available in terms of nutrients per calorie. They are bursting with antioxidants, fiber, important phytonutrients, anti-cancer agents, and vitamins like A and C. They should be a staple of any athlete's diet—served raw or lightly sautéed with garlic.

- **Quinoa**—Quinoa is a South American grain (a seed, actually) that is a complete protein, containing all nine essential amino acids. Dense in fiber and protein and rich in manganese, magnesium, iron, zinc, potassium, and calcium, it's an ideal energy food. Quinoa is usually prepared like pasta and boiled to soften, then added to salads. It can even be used as an oatmeal substitute at breakfast.

- **Almond butter**—Most nut butters are healthful foods, with high protein levels and ample monounsaturated fats. But peanut butter often contains a great deal of sugar. Not so with natural almond butter. It's a great protein and healthy fat source with abundant calcium, fiber, magnesium, folic acid, potassium, and Vitamin E. It's a terrific way to add healthful calories to your training diet.

- **Bananas**—Bananas are portable complex carbohydrates and electrolytes. Wrapped in a neat leaf package, these fruits are ideal for endurance athletes because they are easy to digest, contain a great deal of potassium (which is lost through perspiration), and provide a quick boost of carbohydrate energy.

- **Beetroot juice**—A study at the University of Exeter showed that the natural nitrates in beetroot juice increase the body's levels of NO, relaxing blood vessels and increasing circulatory volume for better transport of fuel and oxygen to muscles. In the study, cyclists drank 500 ml of organic beetroot juice for six days, then were tested for endurance on a cycling course. Versus a control group, the beetroot juice drinkers reduced their time by 2% and also had lower blood pressure readings. Study author Andy Jones said, "Our study is the first to show that nitrate-rich food can increase exercise endurance. We were amazed by the effects of beet-root juice on oxygen uptake, because these effects cannot be achieved by any other known means, including training."

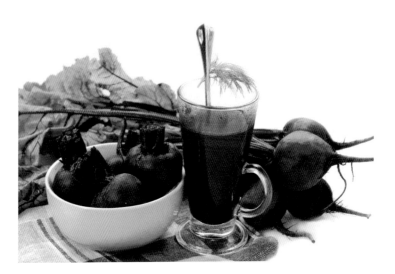

Featured Athlete: Walt Hampton

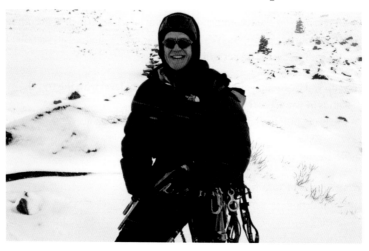

An attorney by profession, Walt Hampton is also an accomplished high altitude mountaineer, distance runner, and wilderness EMT. At 54, he insists he's in better shape than when he was in his 20s and has proven that by summiting mountains all over the world, including his big catch, Denali. He shares his secrets to high-level endurance and recovery:

What is your daily workout routine?

Mondays, Tuesdays, and Thursdays, my wife and I run six miles. Saturdays, we run 14-16 miles or more. Tuesdays, Thursdays, and Fridays, we do Stair-Master or elliptical work (often with backpacks) for 45 minutes to an hour. Mondays and Wednesdays, we do strength and weight training.

What is your typical daily diet?

Breakfast: oatmeal. Lunch: salad. Dinner: salad with shrimp or scallops, a veggie burger, a veggie burrito or veggie frittatas. Snacks: fruit and/or vegetables. Dessert: frozen, low-fat yogurt.

Do you use dietary supplements? If so, which ones?

Multi-vitamin, B-complex, Vitamin D3, Vitamin E, Coenzyme Q10, resveratrol, curcuma, pomegranate, a mitochondrial energy product, and nitric oxide promoting nutrients. I was a single dad for a dozen years, and five years ago, I happened upon a woman who's as crazy as I am. We got married, and we're into living vitally. She read a book that recommended NO. We hooked up with a naturopathic medical doctor who does annual blood testing, and she recommended a regimen of supplements, including NO for supporting nutrition. We've used it now for two-and-a-half years, and it helps with recovery and performance.

How do you maintain your optimal performance level with the travel demands of your sport?

We plan our travel schedule around our training schedule. We always have pre-planned running routes at our destinations. We always stay at hotels with above average workout facilities.

What aspects of your fitness and nutrition program do you consider most important for getting the results you want (e.g., core training for preventing injury, etc.)?

Consistency in diet, consistency in training, and resting.

From a nutritional and exercise perspective, what would you recommend to the young athlete or weekend warrior who wants to take his or her performance to the next level?

Start VERY slowly. Build VERY slowly. Be meticulously consistent. My son was going to give up smoking and said he would run five miles. I said, "Don't do it. Run to the other end of the block and back." People set these huge objectives, feel terrible after they try them, and then don't go out again. Set really conservative goals, and then push it out slowly and consistently. Don't ever push it to where you risk injury. Don't push through because of ego. Listen to your body.

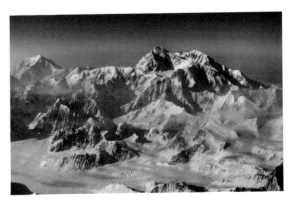

What is your greatest sports moment?

Standing on the summit of Denali, 20,320 feet, after three attempts spread out over nearly 20 years.

What are the top three things you would recommend to a recreationally elite athlete to improve performance as he or she ages?

Be consistent, eat well, exercise, and supplement. I'm in better aerobic and physical shape than I was in my twenties.

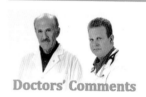

Doctors' Comments

Walt is an exceptional specimen for a man of his age, and clearly, one of the reasons he is able to continue performing at such a high level is his use of NO for supporting nutrition. His high-altitude sport demands strong blood flow, which NO delivers. Recreational athletes and the fitness-minded, who are in or past middle age, would do well, as Walt does, to supplement with a selection of Power Nutrients that both boost and protect NO stores.

Power Nutrients and Endurance

- **Antioxidants**—It is not surprising that hours of distance running, triathlon training, cycling, or skiing can produce excessive levels of exercise-induced free radicals, while depleting the body's antioxidant defenses. The regular intake of antioxidants via daily supplementation has been shown to reduce muscular free radical damage due to exercise, thereby aiding recovery and decreasing the chances of muscular breakdown. As a small range of antioxidants is not sufficient to neutralize all free radicals, it is recommended that endurance athletes supplement with a broad array of antioxidant nutrients such as Vitamins C and E, as well as extracts from green tea, acai berry, goji berry, pomegranate, resveratrol, and alpha lipoic acid.

- **Arginine**—A study published in the *Journal of Applied Physiology* suggests that arginine is an endurance booster. Researchers found that male exercisers taking six grams of arginine as a supplement had a reduced oxygen cost during moderate exercise and greater endurance during intense exercise. Another study at the University of Exeter (where the beetroot juice study occurred) compared athletes taking an arginine supplement with those drinking a placebo black currant drink. The athletes taking arginine showed multiple increases in performance, including a 20% improvement in severe intensity exercise endurance. Because arginine increases the body's levels of NO, improving circulation and transport of nutrients and oxygen, it would stand to reason that this conditionally essential amino acid should be a part of an endurance athlete's regular regimen.

- **Omega-3 fatty acids**—Omega-3 fatty acids have been shown to offer multiple physiological benefits: increased oxygen levels in the bloodstream, improved cardiac function, stronger cell membranes, and, as we have discussed, a reduction in tissue inflammation following intense exercise. For these reasons, endurance athletes, who depend on long-term efficiency of their cardiovascular system for both intense training and performance in endurance events, should supplement with omega-3 fatty acids, generally in the form of fish oil. Vegetarians or vegans who do not wish to ingest fish oil can take flaxseed as a supplement, though it is not as efficient because the alpha linolenic acid in flaxseed must be converted into DHA and EPA, the two fatty acids that comprise Omega-3s. In general, it takes several weeks for Omega-3 fatty acids to saturate muscle fibers, so supplementation should begin well before beneficial effects are needed.

- **BCAA**—These amino acids, which include leucine and valine, have performance-enhancing properties for endurance events, such as marathons, that typically last more than three hours. The reason for this is that as BCAA levels drop, the amino acids are taken up by muscle and serotonin formation increases. This can enhance the athlete's feeling of fatigue, even if glycogen fuel stores and oxygenation are sufficient to continue exercise. A study at Research Laboratories in Stockholm, Sweden, featuring elite endurance cyclists, showed that three grams of a BCAA supplement helped quell this serotonin rise by preventing depletion due to muscular uptake of the amino acids. This also optimized the body's use of available fuel.

- **Glutamine**—Research reveals that intense exercise depletes the body's glutamine levels to the point where catabolism, or muscle consumption, occurs. Endurance athletes can benefit from supplementation with this amino acid to improve glycogen storage, as well as transport, recovery, amino acid synthesis, and prevention of the consumption of muscle fibers. This will enhance performance in endurance athletes of all levels while avoiding injury and weakness caused by muscle breakdown. Supplementation is most effective during periods of high-intensity training, when skeletal muscle and immune function are most at risk.

Power Nutrients for Endurance

- Antioxidants
- L-arginine
- Omega-3
- BCAA
- L-glutamine

Chapter Eight
Nutrition and Recovery

All athletes depend on sufficient recovery to repair damaged muscles, connective tissue, and joints, replenish depleted nutrients, and clear the body of lactic acid and other performance-damping waste products. Many athletes seem reluctant to give recovery its due, perhaps from the misguided thinking that more work is always good. But in reality, recovery is an integral component of the process of athletic training and overall fitness.

Overall, recovery has four components:

1. **Sleep**—Americans, on the whole, do not get enough deep, restorative sleep. This is a problem for the sedentary desk jockey who wants to be more alert; it's a crisis for the finely tuned triathlete hoping to be one of the first off the bike and eager not to pull a hamstring in the marathon. Every active athlete should get at least eight hours of uninterrupted sleep per night. Completing the last workout of the day at least three hours prior to bedtime helps this effort by allowing mind and body to wind down. Sleep allows lactic acid levels to drop, promotes muscle building, rebalances fatigue-inducing hormone levels, and allows your body to properly absorb the nutrients you give it.

2. **Stretching**—Stretching before and after workouts prevents injury, but it is most beneficial when muscles are warm after a heavy exercise program. Stretching lengthens muscle fibers, strengthening them and making them more amenable to the sudden flexion and contraction of power surges in sports like track and field or baseball. It also improves circulation and the function of the lymphatic system, which removes waste from the body. Yoga and Pilates are common

programs for deep muscle stretching and its companion discipline, deep breathing.

3. **Inactivity**—As 2010 Ironman™ World Champion Chris McCormack says in his book, *I'm Here to Win,* you don't get stronger on the bike or at the gym, but on the couch watching TV after your workout. Rest and inactivity—simply refraining from athletic training and letting your body be idle—is essential to effective recovery, especially injury prevention. Many athletes injure themselves in training because they over-train and fail to pay attention to the signals their bodies send: sore muscles, exhaustion, tightness, or joint pain, among others. During rest, the body is working to repair itself from the damage inflicted on it by stressful exercise. This is why most workout programs incorporate at least one day of rest.

4. **Deep muscle work**—Bestselling home exercise programs feature recovery weeks after three or four weeks of rigorous strength and cardiovascular training. These recovery weeks are not idle; they include workouts that engage the body's aerobic and anaerobic systems without pushing the muscles toward injury. In addition, this lighter athletic activity also accelerates the removal of lactic acid from tissues due to increased blood flow. Very effective recovery disciplines include core work, yoga, and deep stretching. Such work keeps the muscles engaged and active, without causing damage. Deep muscle work can also include massage, something that many elite athletes find to be powerfully restorative.

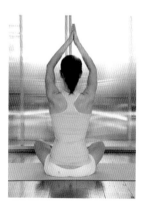

Recovery is the time when the body adapts to the eustress of physical training by developing new muscle mass and restoring the body's glycogen levels. The period directly following an intense workout is particularly important for athletic training. During this time, the body is especially drained and vulnerable to injury and exhaustion. However, it is also primed for the uptake of vital nutrients that can speed muscle repair, bolster the immune system, and jump-start the replenishment of fuel supplies. It is vital that all types of athletes—speed, strength, and endurance—know to give their bodies the proper nutrients during this recovery window of opportunity. Because this is a book about performance nutrition, we will focus on the nutritional aspects of a proper recovery.

Hydration

Although water has no nutritional value, it remains the single most important ingested substance for health and the optimal function of the body. Exercise seriously depletes this vital molecule, so much so that distance runners and other endurance athletes must rehydrate while competing to reduce the risk of cramping, injury, overheating, and dangerous conditions such as heatstroke. After an intense session in the gym, on the track, or on the bike, your body needs water. Most of the water an elite athlete loses will be replenished via supplement and electrolyte drinks, but it is essential to ensure that you do not suffer from chronic dehydration. If you are thirsty during a workout, you are already dehydrated.

The guideline for dehydration during intensive exercise is that you should not lose more than 2% of your body weight via fluid loss. In other words, a 200-pound male running a marathon can finish the race weighing 196 pounds and be within acceptable parameters. During recovery from either training or competition, rehydration becomes especially important. Drink about 16 oz. of water per pound of lost body weight to rehydrate yourself properly. While shakes and other sports supplements designed for recovery are fine for this purpose, avoid the salty, consumer-oriented electrolyte drinks. They are high in sugar and contain none of the antioxidants and other key nutrients your body craves after a hard workout.

Also, be cautious about overhydration during recovery. A 2005 study published in the *New England Journal of Medicine* tracked 488 runners who had completed the Boston Marathon and found 13% of them had dangerously low blood salt levels, a condition known as hyponatremia. This can occur when an athlete drinks so much plain water that vital electrolytes become diluted. Instead of drinking plain water until satiated, it is more prudent to consume nutritional drinks immediately after exercise to restore electrolyte levels, then "top off" with water.

Featured Athlete: Jason Lester, Ultraman, Creator of EPIC5, and the 2009 ESPY Winner for Best Male Athlete with a Disability

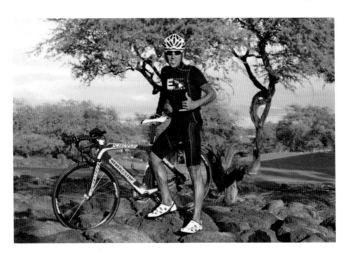

Jason Lester finished the punishing Ultraman triathlon (a double-length, Ironman™ run over three days), ran 306 miles from Las Vegas to California's Mt. Whitney to raise money for clean water, and both created and completed the EPIC5 Challenge—five Ironman™ triathlons on five different Hawaiian islands on five consecutive days. And he's done it all with a paralyzed right arm. Now this incredible endurance athlete, who's also a vegan and the author of *Running on Faith*, shares his secrets for endurance and performance:

What is your daily workout routine?

My daily workout varies, depending on what race I am training for. Normally, I'll do two sessions a day—either a bike/swim or swim/run. I average between 3-4 hours of training a day.

What is your typical daily diet?

For breakfast, the first thing I take when I wake up, before my workout, is an electrolyte beverage. After my workout, I'll have a vegan shake. Hemp and flax oil are standard smoothie additions. For lunch, I'll often eat almond butter with hemp bread and agave or an Avocado-Veganaise® sandwich. Depending on where I'm at with training, I'll have another smoothie or juice with greens in the afternoon. I make it a point to eat fresh fruits and one avocado during the day. A typical dinner would be lots of greens with tofu and brown rice.

Do you use dietary supplements? If so, which ones?

I try and absorb all my vitamins from real foods, but I do take chromium and, sometimes, will take a BCAA (branch chain amino acid) supplement.

What foods do you eat and what supplements do you take to promote recovery, allowing you to train with greater intensity while preventing injury?

I don't take any supplements for recovery since I'm a firm believer that real, plant-based food is the best aid in healing. Being a vegan, everything I eat is plant-based. Another key component for full recovery is rest. I try to fit a nap in between training sessions as often as I can.

Are you familiar with the benefits of nitric oxide? If so, do you incorporate it into your nutritional regimen?

I'm very familiar, but I'm a firm believer that individuals have to choose his/her supplements for themselves. I've been racing and training since I was 15 years old, so I know what works for me. That's why I've chosen a plant-based diet and to be vegan. I try not to venture off into supplements that may work for some people, though not necessarily for me. I continue to use what I know works best for my own performance and recovery. I've also found that, as I've integrated not shying away from oils, avocados, and good fats, it helps with my recovery.

One of the reasons I created my EPIC5 Challenge was that I wanted to see what the human body could accomplish on a plant-based diet. I made it a point to eat only real foods, such as almond butter or avocado sandwiches, and take in electrolytes from natural sources, such as coconut water. Any additional nutritional supplements were from the Vega product line of all natural, plant-based ingredients. My recovery each day was right on target. I didn't need to use gels, bars, or fast-acting sugar products. All sugars came from real fruit and real foods.

How do you maintain your optimal performance level with the travel demands of your sport?

One of the great things about the foods I eat is that they are mobile—smoothies, bars, and supplements. I travel with my blender to make fresh, on-the-go smoothies since it's hard to find optimal nutrition on the road. I like to find out where the local, organic markets are, as well as prepare meals in advance before traveling.

What aspects of your fitness and nutrition program do you consider most important for getting the results you want (e.g., core training for preventing injury, etc.)?

Core training is very high on my list; I incorporate it in my training routine. I also have a specific core routine I do at the gym twice a week. I've seen great results in not just swimming but also running and biking. I'm very much all for core training for performance.

From a nutritional and exercise perspective, what would you recommend to the young athlete or weekend warrior who wants to take his or her performance to the next level?

I feel that any athlete, from weekend warrior or beginner, to advanced, can benefit from incorporating a more plant-based diet into his or her lifestyle, simply because the more real foods we eat, the more alive we'll feel. I've seen great advancement in my training and recovery from going vegan and having a plant-based diet.

What is your greatest sports moment?

My greatest moment would have to be the 2008 Ultraman World Championships in Kona and becoming the first athlete with a disability to finish the race. This earned me my ESPY nomination.

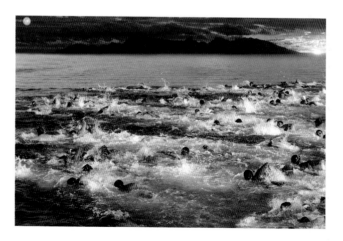

What are the top three things you would recommend to a recreational or elite athlete to improve performance as he or she ages?

Listen and stay tuned in to your body. Your body speaks the truth. It will tell you what it needs. Train smarter, not harder. It's better to be under-trained by 5% than over-trained. It's okay to miss workouts if your body needs to rest. Rest and recovery allow you to train that much harder and stronger the next day. If you're not in tune with your body, you will only break down. Nutrition and rest are two of the most valuable components for performance.

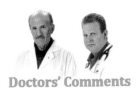

Doctors' Comments

As a vegan endurance athlete, Jason is a rare breed. It is likely that, despite the extremely healthful qualities of his plant-based diet, he does not get all the dietary NO he needs. However, because of his unbelievable level of exercise, it's safe to say his NO production is in the stratosphere. He is also likely to get sufficient antioxidants to help his body recover through his vegan diet. However, for amateur endurance athletes who are not vegan and not training at Jason's level, supplementation is the key to building NO quantities and also getting the antioxidants needed to prevent cell damage in recovery.

NO and Recovery

How *doesn't* NO assist the athletic body in recovery? It helps clear the tissues of lactic acid, reducing fatigue and allowing athletes to get back to work sooner. It promotes improved circulatory volume, which cleanses the body of other waste products. It functions as an antioxidant, preventing free radical damage caused by intense exercise. It acts as an anti-inflammatory agent, preventing some of the pain and swelling that can occur in muscles and joints following training. It delivers nutrients and oxygen to tired muscles, allowing greater gains in size and strength after resistance training.

In short, NO is a "recovery engine." Having optimal stores of it is vital to effective post-activity recovery for all athletes, regardless of whether their sports center on speed, strength, endurance, or a blend of all three. Athletes seeking to avoid post-workout injuries, maximize the muscular and cardiovascular benefits of high-intensity training, and return to their sports more quickly following challenging exercise, would be well-advised to supplement with NO precursors and the nutrients that support this incredible molecule.

Diet and Recovery

The recovery diet should be rich in two macronutrients: complex carbohydrates and lean protein. After you have reduced your body's glycogen stores with a high-intensity workout, it will be demanding the reintroduction of complex carbohydrates to replenish those stores. The body will accept simple sugars, but these have the disadvantage of being digested quickly, spiking insulin levels, and reducing muscle absorption of the glycogen product. Complex carbohydrates, on the other hand, break down slowly, increasing the amount of fuel the muscles can reabsorb.

The difference in performance between an athlete who regularly refuels with carbohydrates immediately after exercising and throughout the recovery phase, and one who does not, can be enormous. Your body has limited on-board glycogen storage; even elite athletes with perfect nutrition can only run or cycle off stored energy for 75-90 minutes. But that is a far cry from a poorly recovered athlete who either refuels at the wrong times or consumes poor quality carbohydrates. Such an athlete might have only 20 minutes worth of fuel in his or her muscles—enough to cover perhaps three miles of a marathon at a moderate pace. Such an athlete will need to carry more nutrition during races, increasing weight, the need to urinate, and the risk of gastrointestinal distress.

The other critical recovery nutrient is protein. As we have discussed, exercise damages your muscles, and protein is the building block of muscular recovery. As micro-tears in muscle fibers heal, they add cellular mass, which becomes new muscle to store additional glycogen. Added muscle translates to added energy and performance. Lean protein sources, as well as protein supplements (see below), are crucial as part of recovery.

For meals immediately following a workout, consume carbohydrates and protein together, as the carbohydrates increase protein absorption. These dietary suggestions reflect the need to combine foods for recovery:

- **Chocolate milk**—This is a surprisingly popular recovery drink! Liquids are popular recovery foods because they are absorbed into the body more quickly than solids. A pint of low-fat chocolate milk has about 300 calories, 50 grams of carbohydrates, and 16-20 grams of protein, making it a perfect start to your post-workout meal.

- **Lean meat and brown rice**—Chicken or steak plus rice delivers a protein punch, along with fiber and complex carbohydrates. Also, the protein/rice combination increases satiety (the feeling of being full) so that you eat only what your body needs to recover and don't consume excess, needless calories.

- **Fish**—Salmon, tuna, tilapia and other white fish are all terrific low-fat, high protein choices. Add a sweet potato or high-carbohydrate steamed vegetable like broccoli or cauliflower to the mix, and you'll get plenty of Omega-3 fatty acids, complex carbohydrates, and fiber to replenish your glycogen stores and rebuild muscles, while muting inflammation.

- **Avocado sandwich**—Avocados are packed with healthful monoun-saturated fats, with a medium-sized fruit containing about 30 grams. This is a calorie-dense food that's great for your cholesterol levels as well as rich in potassium, other trace minerals, Vitamin K, and B-Vitamins. Make your sandwich with whole-grain bread and add complex carbohydrates and fiber to your post-workout meal.

- **Apples with peanut butter**—Again, we're after calorie-rich foods that deliver high levels of healthful nutrients. Apples are not high in calories, but they are nutrient powerhouses, providing pectin, Vitamin C, fiber, and antioxidants. Peanut butter (or other nut butters such as sunflower) contains many needed calories, protein, and beneficial fats.

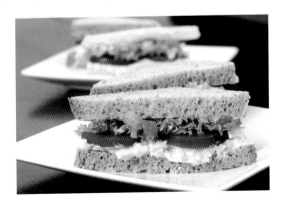

Featured Athlete: George Brett, Retired Major League Baseball Star and Hall of Famer

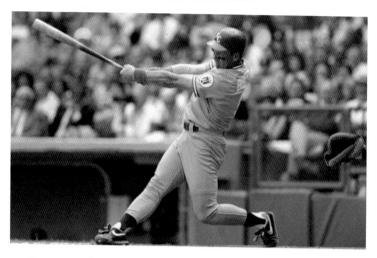

George Brett became a legend during his long career as the third baseman for the Kansas City Royals. Now retired at fifty-eight, he still eats a healthy diet and works out to keep up with his sons and keep himself fit. He shares his secrets to health after a pro career:

What is your daily workout routine?

My workout routine is basically cardio. I do a lot of cardio, ab work, and stretching. I've never really been a weightlifter, although I'm starting to get into it now. But I'd say the average is probably 45 minutes a day, six or seven days a week. I've been to spring training now with the Royals for three weeks, and I've missed one day. So, I'm able to bounce back and work out every day, and I just kind of watch what I eat.

What is your typical daily diet?

I usually take my protein supplements, and mix them with water. I pour a couple of scoopfuls in the shaker; put the top on, shake it up, and drink it right after my workout. I work out at about 9:00a.m. in the morning, so I get done about 10:00-10:15a.m.. I have time for my steam, sauna, and all that stuff.

I have my shake at probably 11:00 or 11:30, and then it's lunchtime. Well, guess what? I go to lunch, and all of a sudden I'm not eating a cheeseburger. I'm not eating a big meal. A lot of times, for lunch, I'll have a salad; I'll have some fish and things like that. I don't go and just pig out. A lot of my friends, when I have lunch with them, will get a burger, a Patty Melt, or a grilled cheese, but they get fries and stuff! And that's one thing that I try to stay away from.

I try to stay away from fast foods, fried foods, and bread as much as possible and just try to eat a lot of protein. You know—fish, chicken, steak. I love them all, and I barbecue a lot. I have three boys in high school who are big boys. They like to eat and they're football and baseball players. So, we spend a lot of time in the summer and winter in Kansas City doing a lot of barbecuing.

Do you use dietary supplements? If so, which ones?

I still take a lot of vitamins—Vitamins B, C, and all that stuff. I think, with all the working out that I do, it's very, very important for me to take the essential vitamins to keep my body in shape. One of the most important things that I take is whey protein powder. I mix it in water after my workouts. I take Coenzyme Q10. I take a lot of Vitamin D along with other multiple vitamins, as well as fish oil, a statin, and baby aspirin I take for my cholesterol.

I think if I didn't take all those things, I wouldn't be able to bounce back the way I do and work out for a minimum of 30 minutes a day per week. I would say the average is probably 45 minutes to an hour. I probably do that five or six days a week. I really believe that, if I didn't take these essential things that my body needs to recover at age fifty-eight, I wouldn't be in as good of shape as I'm in right now.

Once I got a little older, I started taking a lot of protein supplements. And, as a result, I feel better now than I did when I played. I'm 58 years old. I retired at age forty, and, right now, I'm three pounds heavier than when I played.

What foods do you eat and what supplements do you take to promote recovery, allowing you to train with greater intensity while preventing injury?

The older you get, the more your body starts to let you know you're getting older. So, what do you do? You combat it somehow, and I combat it with vitamins and protein. Now, even in my 50s, I have a lot of friends who I played baseball with, and it's amazing how much they work out and all the things that they do to stay in shape. To be able to come back and work out day after day, you have to take these things. I think a lot of people don't know this, but the older you get, the more protein you need.

Are you familiar with the benefits of nitric oxide? If so, do you incorporate it into your nutritional regimen?

I've heard a little bit about nitric oxide and what it does: it increases your blood flow to your muscles, makes your muscles work longer and come back better the next day. If there was a nitric oxide product out there that I believed in, I would definitely take it. To me, it's about rebounding. To me, it's about being able to do something one day and come back and do the same thing the next day. Some days your body is a little sluggish, and with nitric oxide, from what I'm starting to understand, it helps your body bounce back faster. This is better for your muscles, because the oxygen is getting into your muscles. As a result, it's going to keep you bigger and stronger and make you last longer.

What aspects of your fitness and nutrition program do you consider most important for getting the results you want (e.g., core training for preventing injury, etc.)?

The people who work eight to five every day are the people who really have to, in my opinion, take better care of themselves and make better choices. The better choices are taking the daily supplements that you need for your system, watching what you eat, and working out. I know that sometimes when you travel, it's tough to work out. Those are the days that I'm really, really careful what I eat.

Sometimes on a Friday night, I might go out with friends. I might go to a party or a function. I'll put things in my system that I normally don't. But the next day, that's the day that I'll really pound on the treadmill or cardiovascular machines and try to "play for the tie." I think that's why I'm in such good shape, because I have the time and effort to not only watch what I eat, but also exercise daily and make sure I put the right things in my system.

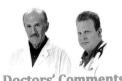

Doctors' Comments

Many professional athletes let their bodies go following the end of their careers. Not this Hall of Famer. George has remained active and fit, and, though he does not supplement with NO, he would benefit from it. His example is illustrative: a middle-aged man with a solid fitness regimen, elevated cholesterol, and a desire to remain well and active for many years. For such men (and women), supplementation with NO enhances recovery, allowing more strenuous workouts, which, in turn, produces greater results. NO has also been shown to have beneficial effects on blood pressure, which can rise in men of George's age. In short, men of almost any age can benefit from NO supplementation as they work to remain fit, vibrant, and healthy into middle age and beyond.

Power Nutrients and Recovery

- **Coenzyme Q10**—Coenzyme Q10 is especially beneficial for the heart, and many patients taking statin drugs also take this Power Nutrient, which is depleted by statins and helps maintain a healthy cardiac muscle. Coenzyme Q10 aids in recovery by helping to optimize the condition of the heart, which helps to increase circulatory volume and pumping power. It also functions as a powerful antioxidant, helping to prevent free radical damage to vulnerable tissues following stressful exercise.

- **BCAA**—Up to 75% of the body's muscle tissue is comprised of these three branched-chain amino acids (leucine, valine, isoleucine), so it's easy to understand how maintaining sufficient levels of BCAA will aid in muscular recovery. They are essential to the muscle building process and should be consumed as part of every athlete's recovery program.

- **Protein**—Whey protein is the gold standard for protein in athletic recovery. Whey isolate protein is the most bioavailable of protein sources, meaning that the body is able to absorb and use a higher percentage of consumed protein from it than from any other protein source, including eggs and soy. Drinking whey isolate shakes is the preferred method for consuming protein post-workout or post-race.

Avoid whey *concentrate*, which usually contains less usable protein and can contain lactose, which many people cannot tolerate.

- **Antioxidants**—Antioxidant supplements containing a broad range of antioxidant nutrients (examples: selenium, zinc, glutathione, Coenzyme Q10 and grape seed extract) are your body's chief defense against the cellular damage caused by oxidative stress. According to some estimates, highly active athletes produce ten times the levels of harmful free radicals as sedentary individuals, through exercise alone, to say nothing of those produced via exposure to environmental toxins, emotional stress, and other causes. Thus, an antioxidant supplement is essential for neutralizing free radicals and preventing damage during recovery.

- **Carnitine**—Carnitine has long been a popular supplement for its performance-enhancing properties, but research now indicates that it can enhance recovery as well. A study published in the *Journal of Strength and Conditioning Research* studied ten men, some of whom took an L-carnitine-L-tartrate supplement, while the others took a placebo. After three weeks of supplementation, the men then engaged in an intensive squat workout. Analysis showed that the men who took the carnitine had lower levels of tissue damage than the placebo group and also had higher levels of a precursor to an important anabolic growth hormone. It appears that carnitine fosters improved muscle repair and growth during the recovery phase.

Power Nutrients for Recovery

- CoQ10
- BCAA (Branched-Chain Amino Acid)
- Protein
- Antioxidants
- L-carnitine

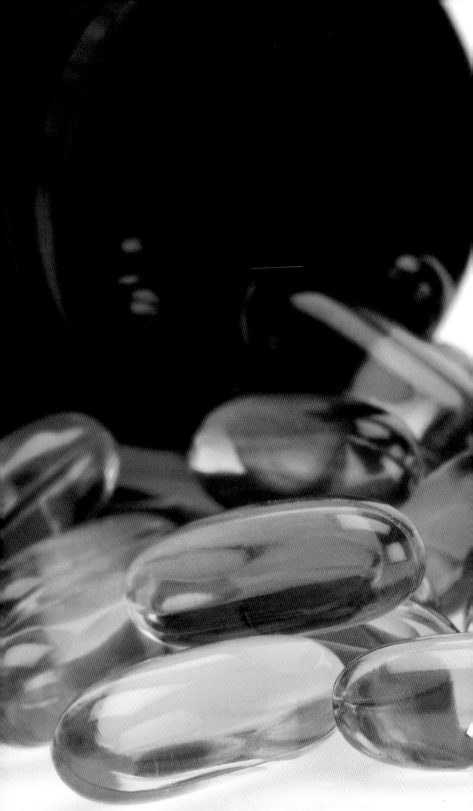

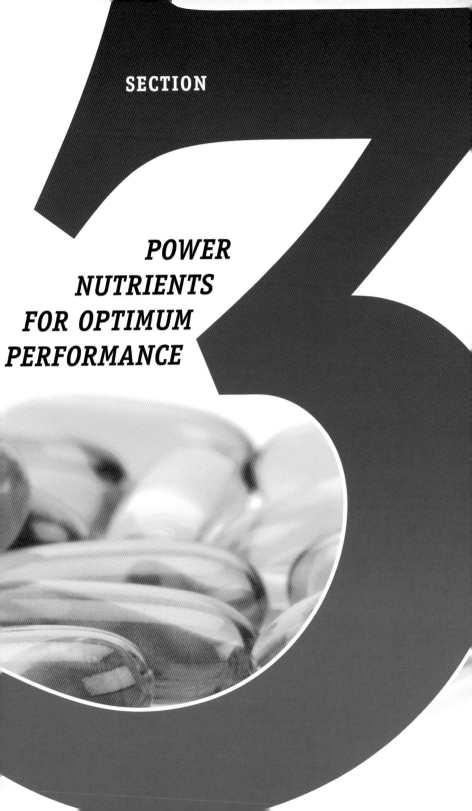

SECTION

3

*POWER
NUTRIENTS
FOR OPTIMUM
PERFORMANCE*

Chapter Nine
Antioxidants

Antioxidant describes a group of nutrients—including vitamins, minerals, and flavonoids—that are effective at neutralizing cell-damaging free radicals. As part of the normal oxidation of food to convert it into energy, free radicals—molecules with unpaired electrons—are formed. Because they have a negative electrical charge, these electrons are drawn to the positively charged protons in nearby cells. This process of "stealing" a proton from a cell's nucleus can cause cellular and DNA damage, possibly leading to cancers and age-related diseases.

What's more, exercise increases the flow of blood to the muscles, which, in turn, delivers more oxygen and other nutrients to the body. As oxygen usage increases, so too does the production of free radicals. You cannot avoid creating free radicals in your body, making protective antioxidants that much more important.

Apart from their other benefits for cardiovascular health, muscle building, and disease prevention, antioxidant-rich foods such as blueberries are full of nutrients that provide elementary particles that pair off with free radicals, preventing them from causing cell damage. Antioxidants appear naturally in many fruits and vegetables, as well as in nuts and grains. Eating a balanced diet that includes a variety of whole fruits and vegetables will help you get a steady supply of antioxidants.

Important antioxidant nutrients include:
- Vitamin E
- Vitamin C
- Selenium (a trace mineral that is required for proper function of one of the body's antioxidant enzyme systems)
- Zinc
- Manganese

In addition to eating foods rich in antioxidants, it is a good idea to increase your intake as part of a daily supplementation regimen, especially when you exercise regularly. Antioxidant supplements can complement your diet as well as keep your antioxidant levels steady during times when you cannot eat your usual balanced diet, such as when traveling for work or competition.

Uses for Athletes

+ Binding to exercise-induced free radicals.
+ Improving blood vessel health through oxygenation of tissues.
+ Enhancing Immune system.
+ Prevention of DNA damage.
+ Optimizing nitric oxide function.
+ Improving exercise tolerance, thereby reducing the impact of post-exercise inflammation and improving recovery.

Antioxidants and Athletic Performance

Dr. Kenneth Cooper, known as the father of aerobics and founder of The Cooper Institute in Dallas, says, "Antioxidant supplements are *mandatory* for adults who exercise."

Dr. Russell Blaylock wrote a book on this subject entitled *Health & Nutrition Secrets That Can Save Your Life*. In his book, Dr. Blaylock writes, "The important thing to remember is that the number of free radicals generated during exercise depends on the intensity of the exercise and its duration. Unless antioxidants in the diet are proportionately increased, intense exercise can actually do more harm than good."

Dr. Rob Childs, nutritional biochemist for a professional cycling team, says that studies dating back to the 1980s have shown that antioxidants reduce muscle damage, while more recent investigations demonstrate that they can also improve both ventilatory and exercise performance. "Such effects are of particular relevance to exercising populations," he says.

Such testimony provides compelling reasons why, if you are a highly competitive athlete who engages in strenuous exercise on a daily basis—training or competition—you should add antioxidants to your nutritional strategy in the form of food, supplements, or both.

Benefits of Antioxidants

Preventing Muscle Damage

The main benefit of supplementation with antioxidants is that it reduces or prevents cellular damage following strenuous exercise. A "cocktail" of antioxidants neutralizes free radical molecules and promotes the healing and growth of muscle tissue during the recovery phase.

Endurance exercise can increase oxygen utilization from 10 to 20 times over the resting state. If you exercise strenuously and regularly, you need antioxidants to help re-oxygenate your body. Otherwise, damage can result. Studies suggest that increased intake of Vitamin E—one powerful antioxidant— is protective against exercise-induced oxidative damage.

Improved Recovery

Many experts in nutritional medicine think that Vitamin E is also involved in the recovery process that follows exercise. Currently, the amount of Vitamin E needed to produce these effects is unknown, but the prevailing opinion is that diet may supply enough Vitamin E for most athletes. We believe supplementation is mandatory with a broad array of antioxidants.

Enhanced Performance

Though antioxidant supplementation has not been proven to be a performance enhancer to the general athletic population, studies do indicate that Vitamin E seems to improve performance in athletes competing in high altitudes. It is suggested that triathletes adjusting to higher elevations may benefit from adding more Vitamin E to their diets. Like Vitamin E, Vitamin C provides benefits in the promotion of nitric oxide's function. Vitamins C and E prevent the oxidation of NO and prolong the lifespan of NO, providing added benefits.

Alpha-lipoic acid (ALA) is a powerful "universal antioxidant" that holds great promise as an "insulin mimicker," aiding in controlling blood sugar levels and the effective use and storage of carbohydrates. ALA's insulin-mimicking affect helps the body store less fat and protect cells from damage. It is also shown to boost the potency of other antioxidants. ALA also potentially reduces muscle fatigue by enhancing the delivery of energy (via glucose and amino acids) into muscles.

Good Dietary Antioxidant Sources

- Green, leafy vegetables, like spinach and kale
- Broccoli and brussel sprouts
- Berries, cherries, red grapes, and Brazilian açai berry
- Cranberries, apples, and strawberries
- Citrus fruits
- Vegetable oils, nuts, and avocados
- Red wine
- Dark chocolate
- Green tea, cinnamon, turmeric, and curcumin

- Radishes and mustard
- Watermelon, guava, and tomatoes
- Squash, apricots, mangos, and carrots
- Grape seed extract

While some foods provide good supplies of antioxidants, you should not depend entirely on food to meet your daily requirements, especially when you are subjecting your body to the stresses of rigorous athletic training. Again, we recommend a combination of supplemental antioxidant nutrition.

Nutrient Connections

The wide and increasing number of antioxidants, as well as the many foods in which they appear, make it impossible to reflect all possible combinations of nutrient interactions here. For more information, please visit www.healthiswealth.net.

Interactions

Note: the majority of prescription and over-the-counter drug interactions with these antioxidants result in reduced levels of the antioxidant in the body, a reaction that is not inherently dangerous. However, check with your healthcare provider before you supplement with antioxidants if you use any of the following medications:

- Vitamin E levels can be reduced by some cholesterol-lowering medications.
- Vitamin C can interact with aspirin and non-steroidal, anti-inflammatory drugs, reducing Vitamin C levels in the body.

Recommended Supplementation

We recommend some combination of the antioxidant nutrients below:

- **Vitamin C**—2,000 to 4,000 mg daily
- **Vitamin E (mixed tocopherols)**—1,000 IU daily
- **Carotenoids (beta carotene)**—25,000 IU daily
- **Zinc**—30 mg daily
- **Selenium**—200 mcg daily
- **Curcumin**—400 to 1,200 mg daily
- **Green Tea Extract**—100 to 750 mg daily of standardized green tea extract (98% polyphenols and 45% EGCG) is recommended. Caffeine-free products are available and recommended if you prefer.
- **Resveratrol**—100 to 200 mg daily
- **Alpha Lipoic Acid**—300 to 600 mg daily
- **Pomegranate Extract**—1,000 mg daily of natural pomegranate polyphenol extract (standardized to 30% punicalagins)

Chapter Ten

Branched-Chain Amino Acids (BCAAs)

BCAA Power Facts

+ BCAAs account for 35% of the essential amino acids in muscle proteins and 40% of the preformed amino acids required by all mammals.

+ Weightlifters and other athletes consuming a higher percentage of BCAAs feel that it is useful for increasing lean muscle mass.

+ BCAAs, like amino acids, do not require digestion; they pass directly into the bloodstream for immediate use by muscle cells.

+ BCAAs provide 70% of the body's nitrogen requirements.

The branched-chain amino acids (BCAAs) leucine, valine, and isoleucine are "chained" together by carbon atoms, and are among the key building blocks of healthy muscles.

Exercise depletes amino acids rapidly, so as an athlete, you must replenish them for your body to function adequately. Failure to do so by an athlete who works out vigorously can cause plateauing and prevent gains in strength, speed, and stamina. A deficiency in BCAAs can also lead to metabolic problems, such as toxicity in the blood and urine.

Making regular gains in physical performance requires regular BCAA replenishment through foods and supplementation. Maintaining sufficient levels of BCAAs also carries with it health benefits such as better brain function, greater muscle strength, and improved endurance.

Uses for Athletes

+ Maintaining plasma levels of key amino acids.

+ Optimizing post-exercise muscle growth.

+ Preventing muscle tissue damage.

+ Improving workout power.

+ Preventing post-workout inflammation.

BCAAs and Athletic Performance

BCAA supplementation has been proven to reduce muscle soreness caused by exercise. In 2009, 12 Japanese long-distance runners between the ages of 19 and 21 participated in a double-blind study for the Saga Nutraceuticals Research Institute to assess the effects of BCAA supplementation on muscle soreness, damage, and inflammation during an intensive training program. The control group was provided placebo supplementation while the remaining participants received the real thing in the form of a beverage.

The result? Those receiving the actual supplementation experienced less soreness and fatigue than the placebo group. In addition, reduced muscle damage and inflammation was also attributed to the effect of BCAA supplementation, which would explain the lower incidence of whole-body soreness.

Given that soreness and plateauing are two of the most common conditions that prevent elite athletes from carrying out intensive training programs and exhibiting ongoing gains in performance, BCAAs must be considered an important supplemental adjunct to any athlete's nutritional strategy.

Benefits of BCAAs

In a recent study conducted by the Department of Life Sciences at the University of Tokyo, it was found that amino acid supplementation affected hematological and biochemical parameters in elite rugby players. According to the study, after just 90 days of supplementation, almost all of the athletes reported improvement in vigor and earlier recovery from fatigue. This is just one of several ongoing studies that point to the benefits of adding regular BCAA supplementation for enhanced athletic performance and greater energy. Other benefits include:

- **Improved recovery**—Most athletes feel a substantial decrease in the amount of muscle soreness after workouts once they begin taking BCAA supplementation. Muscles grow during recovery from the damage caused by pushing them to failure; faster recovery means that you will meet your size and strength goals faster.

- **Enhanced endurance**—BCAA boosts nitrogen in the form of the amino acid L-alanine, which provides the body with a source for the production of glucose after glycogen stores are depleted. Thus, BCAAs may enable you to train at higher intensity levels for longer periods of time.

- **Stimulated protein synthesis**—BCAAs have been shown to induce muscle gains, even in the absence of weight training. Studies have revealed that BCAA supplementation increases levels of testosterone, growth hormone, and insulin.

- **Increased fat loss**—Studies show that supplementation with BCAA triggers significant and preferential losses of visceral body fat (the deeper layer of fat, under the subcutaneous fat, that tends to be resistant to dieting). In one study, 25 competitive wrestlers were divided into one of three diet groups. One group ate a diet high in BCAAs, one ate a diet low in BCAAs, and one ate a control diet. The wrestlers stayed on the diets for 19 days. The high BCAA group lost the most body fat—17.3% of their adipose tissue on average, much of it in the abdominal region.

Benefits of BCAAs

- **Anti-catabolic effects** – By being converted directly into fuel when the body's glycogen stores run low, BCAAs help prevent your body from breaking down muscle proteins for fuel, preventing muscle damage.

Good BCAA Dietary Sources

Dietary sources of BCAA include the following protein-rich foods:
- Dairy products
- Red meats
- Whey
- Eggs

However, while some foods provide BCAA, you cannot depend entirely on food to provide the quantities needed to realize the athletic gains discussed here. Supplementation must complement a varied, healthy diet in order to gain the full range of benefits.

Nutrient Connections
- L-glutamine
- Chromium

Interactions
- None

Recommended Athlete Supplementation
- **L-leucine—500 mg** (2:1:1) 2 to 3 times daily, depending on your workout schedule.
- **L-isoleucine—250 mg** (2:1:1) 2 to 3 times daily, depending on your workout schedule.
- **L-valine—250 mg** (2:1:1) 2 to 3 times daily, depending on your workout schedule.

Chapter Eleven

Coenzyme Q10 (CoQ10)

CoQ10 Power Facts

✦ It's the second most important antioxidant in the cardiovascular system, after nitric oxide.

✦ Statin drugs and aging deplete the body's stores of CoQ10.

✦ CoQ10 is a critical component in cellular energy production in the mitochondria.

✦ Numerous studies have shown supplemental CoQ10 enhances performance.

CoQ10 is one of the most powerful antioxidants in our bodies; it is also vital to boosting cellular energy. Every cell in our bodies relies on an energy source called adenosine triphosphate (ATP), which is produced within the mitochondria (a.k.a., the energy factory) of each cell. CoQ10 assists the mitochondria in transforming food into ATP more efficiently.

Once known as a nonessential coenzyme, CoQ10 is now being classified as an essential fat-soluble vitamin that may potentially protect the body against the harmful effects of free radicals via its antioxidant properties. This nutrient is proving itself as a health booster and a good way to promote heart health.

Uses for Athletes

✦ **Producing energy—CoQ10 is involved in mitochondrial function and the production of energy from fat.**

✦ **Serving as an antioxidant, especially in the cardiovascular system.**

✦ **Benefitting people with obesity, metabolic syndrome, diabetes, cardiovascular disease, immune problems, gum disease, and Parkinson's disease.**

✦ **Attaining positive impact on exercise and sports performance.**

CoQ10 and Athletic Performance

CoQ10 can help athletes maintain energy and improve endurance during exercise by enabling the heart to pump more blood and increasing the ability of tissues to tolerate reduced oxygen levels. CoQ10's positive impact on cardiovascular health and energy levels is why world-class athletes such as 2010 Ironman™ World Champion Chris McCormack take it in supplement form. It is a powerful potential ally for the athlete engaged in a stressful regular training program.

In a double-blinded, placebo-controlled, triple-crossover study, researchers from Japan found that CoQ10 improves athletic performance and fatigue. The researchers recruited 176 healthy adults. The control group received a placebo for eight days, a test group took 100 mg of CoQ10 daily for eight days, and a third group took 300 mg each day for eight days. The men's and women's physical performance was tested using a bicycle ergometer, which measures energy output.

When the study was complete, the physical performance of subjects had increased while they were taking the 300 mg of CoQ10. The subjects also reported feeling less fatigued. This promising study points the way for further research into the effective dosages of CoQ10.

Benefits of CoQ10

Energy Enhancement

CoQ10 enhances energy levels in athletes and non-athletes alike by assisting in the conversion of carbohydrates and fats to energy. The nutrient is necessary for mitochondrial conversion of glucose into adenosine triphosphate, or ATP, the basic energy source of all cells. Optimal CoQ10 levels promote optimal energy production and muscle function.

Improved Performance at Low Oxygen Levels

Where a limited oxygen supply exists (hypoxia), CoQ10 improves the heart's ability to survive and produce energy. Hypoxia occurs at high altitudes, when blood flow is impaired where arteries are clogged, after blood clots, during angina, and when there are high levels of fat in the blood.

Improved Muscle Condition

CoQ10 helps prevent damage to muscles during exercise and increases stamina. A Japanese study showed that athletes taking CoQ10 had fewer markers of muscle damage in their blood after taking the supplement for 20 days than athletes who did not take the supplement. This supports the idea that CoQ10 functions as a powerful antioxidant.

Better Athletic Performance

Studies of CoQ10 supplementation in sedentary individuals and athletes have shown improvement in physical function. CoQ10 has been shown to improve heart rate, workload capacity, and oxygen requirements. These improvements were significant and evident after just a few weeks of supplementation.

Cardiac Health

CoQ10 has been shown in various studies to significantly enhance the heart's ability to pump blood. Research also suggests that supplementing with CoQ10 may even help slow down the aging process and stave off some of its effects. One study, published in the *American Journal of Cardiology*, revealed that heart patients taking CoQ10, either alone or with medications, lived an average of three years longer than those who didn't supplement with the nutrient! This is of particular interest to individuals over the age of 55, who are often found to be CoQ10-deficient.

Benefits of CoQ10

Good Dietary CoQ10 Sources

Natural dietary sources of CoQ10 include fish, organic meat, and whole grains. However, because food can provide only a small amount of the CoQ10 necessary for athletic and health benefits, supplementation is usually necessary to build up the body's stores of this nutrient to sufficient levels. Note also that cooking and processing foods destroys naturally occurring CoQ10.

Nutrient Connections

- Nitric oxide-forming amino acids arginine and citrulline
- L-carnitine
- Omega-3 fatty acids
- Alpha lipoic acid
- Vitamin E

Interactions

- Statin drugs deplete the body of CoQ10.

Recommended Athlete Supplementation

- CoQ10—400 to 800 mg daily

Chapter Twelve

Creatine

Creatine Power Facts

✦ Creatine forms phosphocreatine in the body and is used to make ATP (the energy currency of our cells).

✦ Creatine stimulates protein synthesis and decreases the breakdown of protein within muscle tissue, enabling muscle cells to become larger and stronger.

✦ Creatine has been shown to significantly improve cognitive performance and memory.

✦ Creatine has been used by Olympic athletes to enhance their performance.

A natural amino acid metabolite, also known as methylguanidine and methylguanidino-acetic acid, creatine enhances muscle gain and recovery, boosts energy and endurance, and aids the body in sustaining the high levels of energy that it needs when working out intensely. Perhaps its most vital role is in producing the energy essential for muscular contractions and explosive movements.

Creatine and Athletic Performance

Many athletes find creatine to be a vital part of their nutrient routine, because it helps them train harder for longer periods of time. In turn, this leads to faster muscle growth, greater strength, and enhanced performance. In more than 200 university studies, creatine has been shown to enhance athletic performance and muscle building. It has also been shown to increase gains in lean body mass and boost fat loss.

Furthermore, creatine is demonstrated to have benefits in mental performance. In one study, participants who received eight grams of creatine for five consecutive days experienced dramatically less mental fatigue due to increased oxygen consumption in the brain. When performing numerical calculations, those who supplemented with creatine performed far better after five days than they did before beginning supplementation. While we frequently focus on the function of our muscles during athletic performance, the mind plays a critical role in optimal performance.

Benefits of Creatine

Larger Muscles

Creatine is a cell volumizer, which is good news for fitness buffs and athletes. Intake of creatine and water causes muscle cells to become super-hydrated. In turn, muscles become fuller, and muscle growth is enhanced due to the muscle fibers becoming larger and longer.

Better Sprint Performance

Creatine improves muscle contraction speed and endurance in high-intensity activities that briefly engage the aerobic system, such as sprinting.

Reduced Fatigue

Creatine delays training fatigue, allowing longer muscular contractions by enhancing the cellular energy manufacturing process.

Improved Overall Health

Creatine has been shown in medical studies to promote overall good health by reducing blood lipids (fats, such as cholesterol and triglycerides) that are known to cause heart disease and other adverse conditions. Creatine also appears to improve the metabolism of blood sugar, which can enhance insulin sensitivity and help blood sugar reach the cells faster, helping to combat the development of diabetes, obesity, and heart disease.

New research indicates that creatine may have positive effects on mental performance and even reduce allergic responses by helping reduce the production of histamine.

Other Important Creatine Facts

While creatine monohydrate is the most recognized form of this supplement, alternative forms of creatine are available that offer similar benefits to the monohydrate form. However, each has pros and cons. For example, *creatine citrate* has been shown to reach its peak concentration in the blood within one hour; creatine monohydrate takes up to three hours. Creatine citrate tends to dissolve more easily in water than the monohydrate form, which may indicate that it is absorbed more quickly into the bloodstream.

The downside is that you would need to consume nearly twice as much in grams of creatine citrate to get the same amount of creatine in your bloodstream as you would with the monohydrate form.

Creatine also starts to destabilize after only a few hours of exposure to liquid, leaving a worthless by-product called creatinine. In a 2003 study that compared a creatine serum to a powdered creatine monohydrate supplement, the serum was completely ineffective, performing no better than a placebo. The monohydrate powder increased levels of creatine in the muscles by about 30%.

Good Dietary Creatine Sources

Dietary sources of creatine include:

- Red meat
- Pork
- Tuna
- Herring
- Salmon

The body produces some creatine, primarily in the liver. But while some foods can provide creatine in your diet, you cannot depend entirely on food to provide sufficient levels to gain the maximum muscle-building effects. Eat the right foods while supplementing. Good quality whey or soy proteins (probably ingested in the form of supplement shakes) can aid in creatine uptake, leading to enhanced rebuilding of muscle tissues and prevention of muscle breakdown.

If you train intensely, are involved in rigorous physical activity, or limit your consumption of red meat, you may have low reserves of creatine. It would be advisable to add creatine supplements to your diet and exercise routine.

Nutrient Connections

- Protein
- Alpha lipoic acid
- CoQ10

Interactions

- None

Benefits of Creatine

Recommended Athlete Supplementation

For the best results, creatine should be taken within one hour of an intense workout, along with a simple sugar (example: grape juice). Adding a simple sugar greatly increases the uptake of creatine into the muscle cells by stimulating a natural, mild insulin spike. To get the maximum benefits of creatine, experts recommend taking high levels ("loading") for the first five days and then reducing the dose thereafter.

- Loading dosage—20 to 25 grams daily, divided into 3 to 5 servings throughout the day for 5 consecutive days.

- Maintenance dosage—5 to 10 grams, again depending on body weight, once to twice daily.

Chapter Thirteen

Omega-3 Fatty Acids

Omega-3 Power Facts

+ A Harvard study found that over 84,000 people die each year from a deficiency of Omega-3 fatty acids.

+ Experts estimate that nearly 80% of the population does not ingest enough Omega-3 fatty acids, and this includes most athletes.

+ Our cells are surrounded by fatty envelopes. and Omega-3 fatty acids help keep cell membranes healthy, flexible, and functional.

+ The body uses Omega-3 fatty acids to reduce levels of inflammatory hormones called prostaglandins, while promoting anti-inflammatory hormones.

Omega-3 essential fatty acids are "good" fats that cannot be produced by the body and must be supplied by the diet. They are necessary for many bodily functions and processes. For example, Omega-3s support the cardiovascular, reproductive, immune, and nervous systems.

Our bodies cannot make the three most important types of essential fatty acids—EPA (eicosapentaenoic acid), DHA (docosahexaenoic acid), and ALA (alpha-linoleic acid), all of which are Omega-3 fatty acids—so we must get them from our diets. Omega-3 fatty acids are critical to our overall health. They are shown to decrease hallucinations in schizophrenics, improve symptoms in bipolar and obsessive-compulsive disorder, and improve brain function in Alzheimer's disease and autism. Research also shows that sufficient levels of Omega-3 fatty acids can:

- Improve energy production and mental stamina
- Improve the condition of skin, hair, and nails
- Reduce cellular aging
- Reduce the risk of cancer
- Reduce depression symptoms and elevate mood
- Reduce risk factors for cardiovascular disease
- Improve the response to stress
- Improve endocrine function
- Boost autoimmune function
- Improve reproductive function
- Improve liver and kidney function
- Fight the effects of diabetes
- Improve bone mineral retention
- Improve sleep
- Reduce the symptoms of allergies
- Improve digestion
- Reduce hyperactivity
- Speed learning
- Improve concentration

Uses for Athletes

+ Serving as an anti-inflammatory.
+ Supporting cellular membrane structure and function.
+ Distributing antioxidants.
+ Maintaining joint health.
+ Enhancing recovery.

Omega-3 Fatty Acids and Athletic Performance

For the athlete, the primary impact of Omega-3 fatty acids comes in the reduction of tissue inflammation following a demanding workout or competition. Due to the damage that occurs to muscle fibers during intense contraction, as well as the oxidative damage caused by exercise-induced free radicals, muscles can become inflamed and painful after workouts, leading to injury, joint pain, and slow recovery. This can seriously impair performance and the ability to train for peak athleticism.

By inhibiting the body's inflammatory response, Omega-3 fatty acids reduce pain, swelling, tissue damage, and recovery time and promote muscle tissue healing. They also support cellular structure, helping reduce damage at the microscopic level. System-wide, Omega-3 fatty acids foster an array of health benefits that can aid the active individual or elite athlete, from protecting vision to promoting mood stability.

Benefits of Omega-3 Fatty Acids

Reduced Inflammation

Omega-3 fatty acids are powerful anti-inflammatory agents, diminishing the levels of prostaglandin, a hormone associated with the body's natural inflammatory response. As a result, Omega-3 fatty acids reduce tissue inflammation in muscles and joints following rigorous exercise. This, in turn, reduces pain, swelling, muscle trauma and tissue damage, as well as speeds recovery.

Improved Lung Function

An Iranian study showed that supplementation with Omega-3 fatty acids improved both lung function and volume in athletes. This is due to the anti-inflammatory properties of Omega-3 fatty acids, which reduce inflammation in lung tissues, enabling athletes to draw and expel more air and get more oxygen to the tissues during exercise.

Enhanced Cardiovascular Function

A double-blind, placebo-controlled study done by the University of Wollongong in New South Wales, Australia, revealed that athletes who were given daily fish oil supplements had reduced heart rates and lower oxygen consumption than athletes in the control group.

Benefits of Omega-3 Fatty Acids

More Lean Body Mass

It has been known for some time that Omega-3 fatty acids are effective in weight control. But a study published in the October 2010 issue of the *Journal of the International Society of Sports Nutrition* showed that athletes who supplemented actually had better body composition, reduced body fat, and a higher percentage of lean muscle mass.

Reduced Blood Clot Risk

Omega-3 fatty acid supplements lower the hazard of blood clots such as deep vein thromboses, which are a common problem for runners and other endurance athletes who must often wear compression garments to ensure adequate circulation.

Good Dietary Omega-3 Fatty Acid Sources

Excellent dietary sources of Omega-3 fatty acids include:

- Flax seed oil
- Flax seeds
- Flax seed meal
- Hemp seed oil
- Hemp seeds
- Walnuts
- Pumpkin seeds
- Brazil nuts
- Sesame seeds
- Avocados
- Some dark, leafy, green vegetables
- Canola oil (cold-pressed and unrefined, if possible)
- Soybean oil
- Wheat germ oil
- Salmon
- Mackerel
- Sardines
- Anchovies
- Albacore tuna

Benefits of Omega-3 Fatty Acids

Between 15%-20% of your overall daily calorie consumption should come from essential fatty acids. To determine the number of grams of Omega 3 fatty acids you should consume daily, multiply your total daily calories by 0.15 (0.20 for the high-end of the range), and then divide the result by 9, the number of calories in one gram of fat. This will tell you how many grams of EFAs to consume each day.

However, while some foods provide the essential fatty acids in your diet, you cannot depend entirely on food to provide what your body needs regarding your daily requirements. If you regularly go days without eating fish or oils, then you should be supplementing with EFAs.

Nutrient Connections

- CoQ10
- Arginine and citrulline (nitric oxide synthesis)
- Vitamin E

Interactions

- Omega-3 fatty acids may decrease blood pressure and thin the blood. People taking prescription blood pressure medications and/or anticoagulants should consult with their healthcare providers.

Recommended Athlete Supplementation

- Omega-3—900 mg (EPA: 674/DHA: 253) once or twice daily from high-quality, sustainable fish oil sources.

Chapter Fourteen

L-arginine

L-arginine Power Facts

✦ This essential amino acid is the sole precursor to the synthesis of nitric oxide.

✦ Nitric Ooxide levels tend to diminish with stress and aging, making arginine an important supplement.

✦ Often used as a workout supplement because of its role in increasing blood flow through NO promotion.

✦ Plays a role in immune system support, wound healing, hormone release, and ammonia excretion.

L-arginine is an essential amino acid that supports the immune system, fosters wound healing, helps to remove ammonia from the body, and assists in the release of important hormones. This Power Nutrient is also the sole precursor to the gaseous signaling molecule nitric oxide (NO), which, as we have discussed, has innumerable benefits for the athletic body. L-arginine jumpstarts the production of nitric oxide in your bloodstream, opening the blood vessels to allow for better circulation, thereby improving oxygen and nutrient flow to working muscles.

Uses for Athletes

✦ Enhancing workout performance.

✦ Increasing lean body mass.

✦ Enhancing recovery by improving tissue oxygenation.

✦ Supporting the immune system to prevent the respiratory illnesses commonly experienced by endurance athletes.

L-arginine and Athletic Performance

In a recent study conducted by the University of Exeter, nine healthy males participated in various physical challenges on a cycling ergometer, and their performance was measured. The participants were randomly assigned to take either a placebo or an L-arginine supplement. The study found that the athletes who took the supplement experienced a "striking increase in performance by altering the use of oxygen during exercise."

A new Exeter study follows findings of other research performed at the university, showing that the high levels of nitrate in beetroot juice—which also raises NO levels in the body—has a similar, beneficial effect on endurance. According to the study's authors, athletes using L-arginine could exercise up to 20% longer and improve race times by 1%-2%—a potential improvement of up to nine minutes for a professional triathlete in an Ironman™, which could mean the difference between finishing on the podium versus finishing back in the pack.

Benefits of L-arginine

The vasodilatory effects of L-arginine offer proven benefits for athletes across all sports:

Increased Muscle Mass

Arginine increases muscle protein synthesis, allowing muscles to recover and grow after exercise at an accelerated rate. It also enhances blood flow and nutrient delivery to muscles, further fueling growth of lean body tissue.

Benefits of L-arginine

Greater Energy

Arginine combines with the amino acids glycine and methionine to form creatine. As we have already seen, creatine helps the body produce more energy to power increased muscle contraction and expansion. This enhances muscular endurance and longer performance of intense exercise.

Improved Stamina

As the Exeter study cited earlier indicates, the ability of arginine supplementation to dilate blood vessels and deliver greater levels of oxygen and nutrients to tissues improves endurance, allowing athletes to exercise aerobically for longer periods before experiencing fatigue. As a direct precursor to NO, arginine assists in promoting optimum blood pressure levels for athletes, reducing the work that the heart has to accomplish.

Improved Recovery

Arginine's effect on circulation, along with its ability to enhance immune function and speed up wound healing, enhances tissue repair during the vital recovery phase that follows strenuous training or competition.

L-arginine supplementation has been found to significantly reduce systolic blood pressure and also helps to stimulate and maintain erections.

Good Dietary L-Arginine Sources

L-arginine is found in protein-rich foods, including:

- Coconut
- Milk and milk products
- Eggs
- Pork
- Beef
- Poultry
- Seafood
- Cereals that are oat- and wheat-based
- Chocolate
- Nuts and legumes (particularly soybeans and chickpeas)

Benefits of L-arginine

- Seeds (particularly flax seed and raw lentils)
- Raw onion and garlic
- Tofu (the firmer the better)

However, it is difficult through diet alone to consume enough L-arginine to get the benefits of enhanced NO synthesis. That is why supplementation with this vital Power Nutrient is extremely important for athletes.

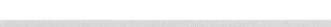

Nutrient Connections

- L-citrulline
- Aspartic Acid
- Glutamic Acid
- Ornithine
- Vitamin C
- Folic Acid

Interactions

- None

Recommended Athlete Supplementation

- L-arginine—5,000 to 1,000 mg daily for optimal performance

Chapter Fifteen
L-citrulline

An organic compound, L-citrulline is necessary for the body's metabolic processes; it helps to maintain the nitrogen balance in the body, which is important in preventing muscle fatigue. Citrulline has been shown to have performance-enhancing effects and to reduce muscle fatigue while boosting metabolic rate. It also helps the immune system fight infection. In a recent study in France, citrulline was found to limit an increase in muscle fatigue that occurs with exposure to bacterial endotoxins.

Uses for Athletes

- ✦ Enhancing performance.

- ✦ Optimizing the removal of waste products during intense exercise.

- ✦ Boosting NO production through recycling into arginine.

- ✦ Preventing muscle fatigue and soreness post-workout or competition.

L-citrulline and Athletic Performance

The effects of L-citrulline on athletic performance have been known (by athletes) for decades. Endurance athletes were using it to help them run farther and cycle longer as far back as the 1970s. L-citrulline was an active ingredient in a product that runners swore by almost four decades ago.

Today, it is experiencing a rebirth of interest among athletes who want to enhance endurance and performance. In a recent study done in Spain, L-citrulline was tested on cyclists. The researchers gave eight young, professional-level cyclists 6 g of L-citrulline, which was a dose equivalent to the total amount of L-arginine that the men consumed daily through their food. Two hours after taking the supplement, the athletes cycled 137 km. Nine other cyclists were given a placebo and made up the control group.

The researchers discovered that the NO levels were boosted in the cyclists who were given the supplement. More nitrite was found in the cyclists' blood immediately after they had finished cycling, as well as three hours later. Nitrite is a marker for NO, which is boosted by ingesting L-citrulline.

Benefits of L-citrulline

The primary benefit of citrulline is that it metabolizes into arginine upon consumption, which, in turn, elevates NO levels and increases dilation of the blood vessels. This results in increased circulation, better oxygen and

Benefits of L-citrulline

nutrient delivery to working muscle tissues, greater muscular endurance, and improved recovery. Other benefits are:

Immune Support

Citrulline helps the body battle fatigue and stress, as well as ensures normal functioning of the immune system. This can be important for endurance athletes who, research has shown, tend to suffer from high levels of respiratory infections immediately following long-distance races, possibly due to the inflammation of lung tissues.

Hormone Production

Citrulline promotes insulin, creatine, and growth hormone production, which helps in muscle building and enhances blood flow.

Increased Aerobic Capacity and Reduced Muscle Fatigue

Taken as the salt citrulline malate, citrulline improves aerobic performance and capacity while it reduces lactic acid metabolism, protecting muscles from fatigue.

Good Dietary L-citrulline Sources

- Watermelon
- Fish
- Meat
- Eggs
- Milk
- Legumes

However, while some foods provide L-citrulline, you cannot depend entirely on food to provide the daily requirements needed for optimal benefits. Supplementation is recommended to enhance performance.

Benefits of L-citrulline

Nutrient Connections

- L-arginine
- Ornithine
- Aspartic acid
- Glutamine
- Proline

Interactions

- None

Recommended Athlete Supplementation

- L-citrulline—1,500 to 3,000 mg daily

Chapter Sixteen

L-glutamine

L-glutamine is a non-essential amino acid (meaning that the body can manufacture it); the liver converts it from the glutamic acid (glutamate) that we ingest. A healthy diet supplies us with the ability to produce between 3.5 and 8 grams of L-glutamine each day. It is the most abundant amino acid, present in all organs. Glutamine promotes optimal organ function and is important to a healthy gastrointestinal tract.

Uses for Athletes

✦ Increasing muscle mass development.

✦ Reducing muscle tissue breakdown during stressful exercise.

✦ Stimulating cell volumizing, which encourages muscle growth.

✦ Enhancing immune function.

✦ Increasing human growth hormone levels.

L-glutamine and Athletic Performance

Athletes who participate in sports that require strength, speed, and endurance use glutamine to help them increase or maintain muscle mass, especially during times of intense training. Extreme endurance athletes, such as marathon runners, benefit from glutamine supplementation, which helps reduce muscle tissue breakdown and supports the immune system during periods of trauma or stress.

L-glutamine is involved in more metabolic processes than any other amino acid. It can be converted to glucose and used as an energy source, which is important for athletes who need energy at the end of a competition or rigorous workout but want to avoid burning muscle tissue. It reduces recovery time after exercise and also reduces healing time following an injury.

For athletes for whom over-training is an issue, such as endurance athletes, rest and L-glutamine can help mitigate the impact of heavy training, while allowing muscles to recover quicker without damage. L-glutamine achieves this through the following mechanisms:

- Building protein within muscles
- Preventing the body from consuming lean tissue for energy
- Restoring glycogen levels, which increases performance

Benefits of L-glutamine

L-glutamine fuels the cells that line the intestines and white blood cells. Without it, immune function can be compromised. It also helps maintain proper function of the kidneys, pancreas, gallbladder, liver, and other organs involved in digestion and elimination. Additional benefits are:

Maintaining Muscle Mass

L-glutamine helps athletes increase or maintain muscle mass, especially during times of intense training. It is often used to help burn victims and surgical patients regenerate tissue at a faster rate, and it has properties that prevent the breaking down of muscle by the body for energy, a process called *catabolism.*

Improved Muscle Growth and Recovery

This supplement stimulates cell volumizing (adding water to the muscle cell), which makes muscles appear larger. It effectively transports amino acids into muscle cells to improve exercise recovery.

Boosted Immune Function

When you train at high intensity or frequency, you risk immune suppression and infections. By supplementing with BCAA, you help reverse glutamine loss. Glutamine is essential for good immune system function.

Increased Mental Clarity

This amino acid operates as a neurotransmitter and also increases blood levels of glutamic acid, which is the primary energy source used by the brain. It is proven to improve mental alertness, clarity of thinking, and mood, and is vital for the endurance athlete at the end of a long, exhausting race.

Good Dietary L-glutamine Sources

- Meat
- Dairy
- Other protein-rich foods

For vegetarians or vegans, as well as those who simply cannot consume enough animal proteins to get a sufficient amount of L-glutamine to reap its benefits, supplementation becomes essential. For athletes, a supplemental L-glutamine regimen is highly recommended.

Nutrient Connections

- Glutamic Acid
- Vitamin B6

Interactions

- No drug interactions are known to exist with L-glutamine. However, simple sugars consumed with L-glutamine after a workout may help transport it into the muscle cells faster and potentially improve recovery. It may be best to supplement with L-glutamine without other amino acids, as it appears to compete with the others for uptake. There is no known toxicity with this supplement.

Recommended Athlete Supplementation

- L-glutamine—5 to 15 mg daily

Chapter Seventeen

L-carnitine

L-carnitine Power Facts

✦ L-carnitine's primary function is to foster the process that turns stored body fat into energy.

✦ Its concentration diminishes as we age.

✦ Carnitine helps maintain bone mass.

✦ Carnitine is also a powerful antioxidant, especially in the heart muscle and endothelium.

Carnitine is derived from two amino acids, lysine and methionine, and its primary function is to foster the process that turns stored body fat into energy. Its beneficial effects on the heart muscle mean that it is commonly used to treat patients with heart failure and angina, but it has numerous uses in the athletic realm that are only now beginning to come to light via clinical research.

Uses for Athletes

✦ Maintaining and improving bone density.

✦ Preventing oxidative damage to the cardiovascular system following exercise.

✦ Boosting dietary energy production at the mitochondrial level.

✦ Enhancing athletic endurance and delaying fatigue.

Carnitine and Athletic Performance

Carnitine plays a vital role in the metabolism of lipids (fats) into energy. This is particularly important for endurance athletes who, during the course of long races, will draw on stored body fat for energy as blood glucose and muscular glycogen are exhausted. Sufficient levels of carnitine ensure that the essential components of lipid metabolism are present to allow stored fat to be converted into usable energy.

Based on a growing body of clinical research, carnitine also plays a central role in effective post-exercise recovery. It appears to do so by reducing the oxidative stress that occurs when athletes exercise strenuously and produce high levels of free radicals. Carnitine also causes those consuming it to reduce abdominal fat and retain more lean body mass. Via this same path, carnitine also reduces muscle soreness and trauma after rigorous exercise.

Given the critical nature of the recovery process, both in pre-event training for competitive athletes such as triathletes, and for the fitness-minded such as bodybuilders, cyclists, and boxers, carnitine is a crucial Power Nutrient. It can increase both the body's recovery time and the level of that recovery, as well as reduce long-term damage from free radical production.

L-carnitine Benefits

Increased Energy Efficiency

Numerous studies have indicated conclusively that carnitine supplementation improves the metabolism of stored body fat into energy during sustained low-intensity exercise such as marathon running or cross-country skiing. This spares glycogen stored in muscles, allowing endurance athletes to perform for greater lengths of time without consuming additional fuel. In a recent 24-week study, athletes who received carnitine supplementation utilized 55% less glycogen while cycling than the control group did. This points to a powerful benefit for athletes in endurance sports.

Improved Recovery

Based on repeated trials, it is clear that carnitine acts as a powerful antioxidant, lowering post-exercise oxidative damage. A double-blind, placebo-controlled study published in August 2010 in the journal, *Metabolism*, revealed that carnitine supplementation in men and women resulted in dramatically lower post-exercise chemical markers of metabolic stress, muscle soreness, and muscle damage than in the control group. This is a clear indication of carnitine's antioxidant power.

Multiple published studies have shown similar results, leading the authors of one study from the University of Connecticut to conclude, "These findings support our previous findings of L-carnitine in younger people that such supplementation can reduce chemical damage to tissues after exercise and optimize the processes of muscle tissue repair and remodeling."

Reduced Lactate Buildup

As we have discussed, the buildup of lactic acid in muscles, due to exercise intensity that exceeds the so-called "lactate threshold," is regarded as a major cause of fatigue and muscle failure. Several studies have examined the role of carnitine in reducing blood lactate levels after high-intensity cycling and found significant improvements. This indicates the strong potential that carnitine, possibly by the same pathways that govern its regulation of fat metabolism, can positively impact the accumulation of lactic acid in the bloodstream and tissues, thereby helping athletes stave off fatigue.

Good Dietary L-carnitine Sources

Red meat (particularly lamb) and dairy products are the primary sources of carnitine. It can also be found in:
- Fish
- Poultry

L-carnitine Benefits

- Tempeh
- Wheat
- Asparagus
- Avocados
- Peanut butter

Nutrient Connections

- Lysine
- Methionine
- Vitamin C
- CoQ10

Interactions

- None

Recommended Athlete Supplementation

- L-carnitine—2,000 to 4,000 mg daily

Chapter Eighteen

Protein

Protein Power Facts

✦ The body contains more than 10,000 different proteins.

✦ Athletes need more protein in their diets than most people.

✦ Proteins are the fundamental chemical building block of body tissues.

✦ Proteins regulate hormone levels.

✦ Protein cannot be stored; it is continually being broken down and must be replenished daily.

Protein is vital to every cell in the body. Our bodies use protein for a variety of purposes: to build and repair tissues, to make enzymes, hormones, and other chemicals in the body; and to form bones, muscles, cartilage, skin, and blood. In short, protein is critically important—in the right portions.

In times of high demand—when we are growing, during pregnancy, and during periods of intense exercise—we need more protein. Protein is the building block of muscles and is essential for repair and growth of muscle after exercise. Particularly during resistance exercise, you cause microscopic damage to the myofibrils of muscle fibers. The body responds to this damage by sending nutrients, including protein, to the muscle to help it grow.

Uses for Athletes

✦ Maintaining muscle growth and during training.

✦ Repairing and rebuilding muscle in recovery.

✦ Boosting metabolic rate.

✦ Preventing or delaying exercise-induced fatigue.

Protein and Athletic Performance

Research suggests that individuals performing endurance activity require more protein intake than sedentary individuals, so that muscles broken down during endurance workouts can be repaired. According to a 2006 nutrition study, endurance athletes can benefit from increasing protein intake, because endurance exercise alters the protein metabolism pathway.

The overall protein requirement increases because of amino acid oxidation in endurance-trained athletes. Endurance athletes who exercise for a long time period (two to five hours per training session) use protein as a source of 5%-10% of their total energy expended. Therefore, a slight increase in protein intake may be beneficial, because it replaces the protein lost in energy expenditure and repairing muscles. Some scientists suggest that endurance athletes should increase daily protein intake to a maximum of 1.2–1.4 grams per kg of body weight.

Research also shows that protein consumed before exercise and within 30 minutes of finishing a workout helps with growth and recovery time. The guideline for protein consumption after exercise is one gram for every 3-4 grams of carbohydrates (for example, two tablespoons of peanut butter has 9 grams of protein). Consult with your dietary or healthcare advisor to help you determine the right amount of protein for your exercise level and competitive needs.

Protein Benefits

Muscle Growth and Development

Protein is the basic chemical building block for muscles, tendons, organs, and most other body tissues. Supplementation with whey protein or other high-quality proteins is proven to increase muscle growth following resistance workouts and prevent muscle loss due to breakdown as the body consumes muscle tissue for energy.

Enhanced Recovery

Research has shown that athletes who consume protein after a hard workout or competition experience less soreness and are able to resume rigorous training sooner than athletes who do not consume supplemental protein through diet, drinks, or other sources.

Improved Glucose Transport

Protein may aid in enhancing glycogen replacement after exercise by stimulating the action of insulin, which transports glucose from the blood into the muscles.

Improved Endurance

Protein supplements have been shown to deliver branched-chain amino acids (BCAAs) to muscles with greater efficiency. BCAAs have been shown to delay the depletion of muscle energy when consumed before and during strenuous exercise, allowing athletes to exert themselves longer.

Weight Loss

Metabolizing protein requires twice as much energy as converting the same quantity of carbohydrates or fat into glucose. The extra effort can increase resting metabolism, or basal metabolic rate, and lead to weight loss in the long term. In the short term, a high-protein diet can also lead to weight loss. According to Frank Hu, M.D., Ph.D., assistant professor in the Department of Nutrition at Harvard University School of Public Health in Boston, while no one knows the effect of eating a high-protein diet over the long term, the diet appears to be safe and effective for up to six months.

Good Dietary Protein Sources

It is possible for athletes to consume enough protein through dietary sources alone. However, the quality of the protein is crucial. Ideally, protein sources should be low in fat and be *complete* proteins, containing all the essential amino acids. For vegetarian or vegan athletes, most non-animal protein sources are *incomplete*, meaning that they are missing some essential amino acids. For non-meat eaters, it is important to properly combine dietary proteins, in order to give the body all the amino acids it needs to form and repair tissues. Common dietary protein sources are:

- Red meat
- Chicken, pork, and fish
- Beans and legumes
- Soy and nuts
- Whole grains
- Peanut butter
- Seeds
- Tofu
- Yogurt
- Milk and soy milk
- Cheese
- Eggs

Unless you are an elite athlete doing tremendous amounts of aerobic or resistance exercise, you probably do not need a protein supplement. Most of us get enough protein in our diet each day. Excess protein is not used by the body; it is excreted in urine. Athletes who work out every day will often require extra protein to fuel muscle growth and rebuilding. Supplementation, which usually occurs in the form of shakes containing whey, rice, and/or soy protein, is calculated based on body weight in kilograms.

Nutrient Connections

- Healthy carbohydrates and fats

Interactions

- None

Recommended Athlete Supplementation

General protein requirements are as follows:
- Adult men need about 56 grams per day.
- Adult women need about 46 grams per day.

Another way to calculate protein requirements is as a percentage of calories. The USDA suggests that protein should make up 17%-21% of total calories. The Institute of Medicine recommends we get at least 10% and no more than 35% of calories from protein.

Athletes may require quite a bit more than the levels above to support muscle repair, increase growth, and protect against the general hardships of vigorous training and competing.

Generally, we suggest no more than about twice the daily recommended protein allowance applicable to less active people.

For endurance athletes, a protein intake of 1.2-1.4 g/kg should be consumed; for strength athletes, 1.2-1.8 g/kg should be consumed. Additional research has shown that endurance athletes actually need more protein than strength athletes due to greater caloric expenditure.

Chapter Nineteen
Simple Health Value

In summary, the philosophy behind *Health is Wealth: Performance Nutrition* is a simple and positive one: you have control over how you tap into your athletic potential. In truth, we do not all enjoy the same athletic gifts. There are individuals who are blessed with a genetic makeup that grants them exceptional speed, body control, coordination, throwing arm strength, or agility; these people often become professional athletes, the elite of the athletic spectrum. However, all human beings possess the potential to maximize their inherent athletic gifts and perform to the utmost limits of their ability. No matter what your athletic genetic inheritance is, you have some control over how your genes express themselves, how your body changes as a result of athletic training, and how you perform competitively. Your success will be determined largely through the lifestyle choices that you make.

It is no secret that, in this book, we promote supplementation as one of the most important positive lifestyle choices. Taking in key Power Nutrients via dietary supplements (as an adjunct to whole foods) is a simple, cost-effective, and empowering way to combat nutrient depletion and deficiency. It's not surprising that 68% of Americans say they take dietary supplements over the course of a year, according to the Council for Responsible Nutrition. If you are taking supplements, are you taking the right balance to enhance your athletic performance and overall wellness? That's a question for you, your coach or trainer, and your healthcare provider to decide. But let us suggest this: if the people you trust with your health and performance disagree with the concept of supplementation as part of the path to improved wellness and a higher quality of life, perhaps it's time to find a more enlightened team.

As we hope we have demonstrated, the vast repository of scientific research supports the idea that Power Nutrient supplementation can give the athletic body what it needs to gain strength and speed, perform well during grueling endurance events, and recover effectively. As you consider what we've said in this book and look at possibly beginning your own Power Nutrient supplementation program or revising the program you're on now, we recommend taking the following steps:

1. **Do your own research.** Don't take our word for it. Doctors and dieticians don't know everything, even Nobel Laureates. Sometimes, timely research brings to light facts that your healthcare provider isn't aware of. Get online and start digging.

2. **Examine your diet**. Are you eating a wide range of whole foods? If you're trying to gain muscle, are you taking in enough calories? If you're in training, are you eating enough? How can you improve your diet?

3. **Look at your rest habits.** Are you getting enough rest between workouts? Are you taking in the nutrients that fuel recovery? Be sure to discuss your recovery plan with your coach or trainer.

4. **Talk to your healthcare provider about injuries or conditions you're likely to encounter as an athlete as you age**. Should you be stepping up your intake of a nutrient because you're over 50? Should you cut back on one or more?

5. **Be careful of hype.** Especially online, a lot of unqualified people make a lot of outrageous claims about "natural" supplements. Just because something is natural doesn't mean it works or that it's good for you. Take claims with a grain of salt and demand solid scientific evidence to back them up.

It's Not Magic

Here's something else to keep in mind: Even if you develop a custom supplement cocktail to suit your athletic pursuits and start taking it right now, you're not going to notice miraculous results overnight. You won't suddenly be able to bench-press 100 lbs. more than before, set a new personal record in your Ironman™ time, or be able to do 30 pull-ups, when you currently struggle to do three. Power Nutrients don't work like that. The *Health is Wealth* strategy is a long-term one designed to reverse the oxidative damage, nutrient depletion, and joint and muscle injury you've inflicted after years of running, rowing, climbing, swinging, or skating. The goal is to replenish the nutrients your body cries for, so that, over months and years, you notice measurable improvements in your performance and well-being. If you're consistent and patient with your supplementation, over time, you will notice that you can run faster, work out longer, and feel better.

In the same vein, we promote a concept that we call "Simple Health Value" as a companion philosophy to our Power Nutrient approach. From this perspective, ensuring optimal athletic performance, as well as vibrant wellness for years and decades, is based upon your entire lifestyle and the choices you make. Nothing in the body exists in isolation. You cannot embark on a Power Nutrient program, eat junk food, stop exercising, and expect to reap any benefits. Your unhealthy choices will effectively cancel out your good choices. No nutrient is powerful enough to counteract poor lifestyle choices. So, if you truly want to maximize your athletic abilities, feel the best you've ever felt in your life, and keep on doing the sports you love well into your 70s, 80s, and beyond, you may need to change everything about how you live—how you eat, sleep, move, play, and deal with the pressures of life. Fortunately, there's a way to do this, and it's much simpler than you might think. It's also cheap, which is vital in this day and age.

Simple Health Value

The Simple Health Value concept is based on five basic principles:

1. Drink 8-12 8 oz. glasses of water every day.
2. Eat fresh food.
3. Move daily.
4. Get more rest.
5. Breathe deeply every day.

What makes this approach unique and effective is that it doesn't take anything away from you. That's revolutionary. We could wag our fingers at you and tell you to stop smoking or give up bacon double cheeseburgers, and, in all honesty, you'd probably be healthier if you did so. But if you're already doing those things, are you going to quit because we scold you? Not likely. One of the most certain roads to failure while counseling people about making lifestyle changes is to tell them all the things they're doing wrong. Nobody likes that. Many just get stubborn and dig in their heels, which helps no one.

So, we are treating you like a grown-up. Simple Health Value isn't about what you give up; it's about adding five good habits to your life. The odds are that, if you're an active athlete, you're already doing some, or all, of these things…but aren't there some that you could be doing better? Do you really get enough sleep each night? Are you drinking mostly sports drinks or soda during the day, rather than water? Do you breathe deeply at any time except when you're training or competing? Most of us could do better at some of these five habits. Over time, as adding beneficial behaviors to your routine helps you perform, look, and feel better, you'll probably do away with some unhealthy habits on your own. After all, the only way that lifestyle changes last is when you choose to make them a priority. So, as you think about how you can make use of the Power Nutrients, remember the five aspects of Simple Health Value:

1. Drink 8-12 8 oz. glasses of water every day. Water is still the best liquid you can put into your body. You might favor electrolyte drinks for rehydration after a workout or during a run, or protein drinks to help with recovery, but always add in plenty of clear water. There are two big reasons. First, drinking water right before a meal makes you feel fuller with no added calories, so you eat less and, over time, lose weight. That's important for most competitive athletes. Secondly, water keeps your kidneys functioning optimally to help clear your body of all the protein that you're taking in as part of your training.

2. Eat fresh food. Primarily, this means consuming more fresh fruits and vegetables daily, along with whole, raw nuts, seeds, and legumes. Simple Health Value is not about cutting certain foods out of your diet. It's about eating a snack of baby carrots while you're at your desk, adding blueberries to your morning oatmeal, eating a handful of raw almonds as a pre-workout pick-me-up, or putting away a huge salad as part of your post-workout meal. The idea is to introduce as much whole, unprocessed food into your body as possible, in part by getting you to "shop the perimeter" of the grocery store. That's where they keep the real food: the produce, dairy, fish, and poultry. The more you stay out of the central aisles where they keep what *The Omnivore's Dilemma* author Michael Pollan calls "edible food-like substances," the better.

Organic food is great, and what's grown in your own garden is best, but, whatever the source, try to add 4-6 servings of fruits or vegetables to your diet every day—the more variety, the better. You'll be getting Power Nutrients, and you'll also load up on the fiber, phytonutrients, and other compounds that help Power Nutrients work even better.

3. Move daily. You probably already do this. As an athlete, whether you're a pro, collegiate athlete, workout fiend, weekend softball player, or mountain biker, you probably get up and get your heart racing more days than not. So we're preaching to the choir a bit here, but bear with us. The fact is, many people, even athletes, don't engage in a *balanced* movement regimen. We're talking about cardiovascular work, resistance training, core work, and flexibility training. Combining all these disciplines works the entire body and contributes to overall wellness. It's a common misconception that if you want to lose weight, you should focus on cardiovascular activity. But did you know that intense strength training actually burns more calories, and that, the more muscle you build, the more calories your body burns just doing its daily business?

Many athletes focus exclusively on the type of training that applies to his or her favorite sport. If you're a professional, we're not going to suggest that you do otherwise. But odds are, you're not. In that case, a program of strenuous movement that builds lean muscle, sculpts your core, strengthens your cardiovascular system, and increases the suppleness and injury resistance of your muscles can only help you in your athletic pursuits. It will also make you stronger and healthier in the long run.

4. Get more rest. This isn't just about sleep, although it could be: the National Sleep Foundation says that 70 million Americans suffer from some sort of sleep disorder. But we're also talking about rest—that mental downtime during which we're awake but resting our minds and senses—not checking our smart phones or updating our Facebook pages. Rest and sleep are enormously important mechanisms for coping with stress, and, for athletes who train regularly, they are vital to your body's ability to repair muscle damage and avoid injury.

The Simple Health Value prescription for rest is an easy one: make downtime and sleep priorities. That's not always easy; too often in our culture, we make sleeplessness into an act of heroism, as though depriving ourselves of that which replenishes our bodies and minds is something to be proud of. But it's actually a sure way to hamper mental performance, increase the risk of injury, and exacerbate the long-term effects of emotional stress and the oxidative stress of exercise. Instead of celebrating insomnia, we recommend carving out sleep and rest time as best you can and also creating your own sleep routine. Make sleep something sacred, with its own space and pre-sleep ritual. Keep to a consistent bedtime and waking time. Clear your bedroom of all screens, from TVs to tablet computers. Create an environment conducive to slumber. As for rest, find 15 minutes a day for quiet meditation, a walk in nature, or daydreaming. Rest allows the brain to rest and replenish important neurochemicals, and can enhance well-being and concentration.

5. Breathe deeply every day. How are you breathing right now? Until you caught a deep breath upon reading that sentence, you were probably breathing shallowly. We're usually unaware of our own breathing, but most of us breathe shallowly most of the day. Shallow breathing reduces the body's oxygen levels and increases the stress response. When you breathe fast and shallowly, your body interprets this to mean that something stressful is happening, and the fight-or-flight response kicks in. Over the long term, the release of the powerful hormones associated with the "stress response" can do serious damage to the body.

When you're training, you're probably breathing deeply, which puts you ahead of most other people. But even when you're not on the exercise bike, running, or lifting, you can benefit from conscious deep breathing. It's one of the best ways to reduce the effects of stress and bring on a feeling of well-being. Try taking a series of deep breaths—inhaling for an eight-count, then exhaling for an eight-count. See how you feel? Breathing is the only autonomic nervous function over which we have any control. Breathing slowly and deeply reduces the body's stress response. It engages the parasympathetic nervous system, which reduces blood pressure. Everything relaxes. This is why products designed to treat hypertension by teaching people to breathe deeply have been approved by the FDA—they work.

A Potent Combination

Imagine what would happen if you took your already healthy athlete's lifestyle and combined it with Power Nutrient supplementation and the five Simple Health Value steps. You would be doing virtually everything possible to ensure that you reach your maximum athletic potential, while giving yourself a huge head start toward a lifetime of vibrant, active wellness. You would improve your odds of avoiding debilitating disease and being able to engage in the activities you love for decades to come. All it takes is a choice.

You realize that when all the cells in all the systems in your body—cardiovascular, muscular, nervous, skeletal, digestive, lymphatic, endocrine, and so on—are conditioned by physical training and have the nutrients they need to respond instantly to your athletic demands, you'll attain maximum possible output for the maximum possible time.

We've given you the information. You already have the athletic drive and passion. The rest is up to you. Health really is wealth, and athletic performance is accessible to everyone. Even if you can't be an Olympian, you can be a champion. Give your body what it needs to perform at its best, and the sky is the limit.

Share Your Optimal Performance

As an athlete, you demand optimal performance from your body. You may think you have achieved it because you look good and have no excess body fat. That's great, but unless you understand how nutrition, NO, and exercise combine to make every cell in your body work like a finely tuned machine, you're leaving greater speed, power, or endurance on the table.

When you're at your peak, muscles put out additional energy to push pedals or lift barbells. Heart and blood vessels transport more oxygen to working muscles. The pancreas secretes just the right level of insulin to help you turn sugar into energy. The stomach, liver, and intestines extract more vital carbs, proteins, and minerals from gels, energy bars, and electrolyte drinks. Peak performance is about your body doing everything you ask it to when you ask it—and sometimes exceeding what you thought were its limits.

The challenge you can give yourself is to track your performance and observe how your results change as you alter your diet and add Power Nutrients (shown in Section 3 of this book) to your supplementation program. We are confident that over time, as you take these steps, you will notice tangible and substantial improvements in whatever measure of athletic optimal performance you're most interested in, from vertical leap to swimming speed to distance off the tee.

Get a clear measure of where you are today in your athletic performance, write it down, apply what you learn from this book, and seeing how far you can take your performance once you understand proper nutrition and the benefits of optimal supplementation.

As you measure your results, please keep us updated by emailing us at **performancenutrition@healthiswealth.net**. Let us know if it's okay to share them with the world and we'll post some of these results on **healthiswealth.net**. Better yet, send us a photo of you in competition or during your daily workout.

Endnotes

Chapter 5

Ian McDonald, "Sugars for Success?" *British Journal of Sports Medicine* 24, no. 2 (1990): 93-94

"Carbohydrate Needs," Masters Athlete, http://www.mastersathlete.com.au.

"Manganese," Micronutrient Information Center, Linus Pauling Institute, Oregon State University.

Anni Heikkinen, Antti Alaranta, Ilkka Helenius, and Tommi Vasankari, "Use of dietary supplements in Olympic athletes is decreasing: a follow-up study between 2002 and 2009," *Journal of the International Society of Sports Nutrition* 8 (2011).

Richard J. Bloomer and Allan H. Goldfarb, "Anaerobic Exercise and Oxidative Stress: A Review," *Canadian Journal of Applied Physiology* 29, no. 3 (2004): 245-63.

O.-C. Skare, Ø. Skadberg, and A.R. Wisnes, "Creatine supplementation improves sprint performance in male sprinters," *Scandinavian Journal of Medicine & Science in Sports* 11, no. 2 (April 2001): 96-102.

Richard J. Bloomer, Douglas E. Larson, Kelsey H. Fisher-Wellman, Andrew J. Galpin, and Brian K. Schilling, "Effect of eicosapentaenoic and docosahexaenoic acid on resting and exercise-induced inflammatory and oxidative stress biomarkers: a randomized, placebo controlled, cross-over study," *Lipids in Health and Disease* 8 (2009): 36.

E.E. Noreen, M.J. Sass, M.L. Crowe, V.A. Pabon, J. Brandauer, L.K. Averill, "Effects of supplemental fish oil on resting metabolic rate, body composition, and salivary cortisol in healthy adults," *Journal of the International Society of Sports Nutrition* 7, no. 31 (2010).

Amir Lerman, MD; John C. Burnett, Jr., MD; Stuart T. Higano, MD; Linda J. McKinley, RN; and David R. Holmes, Jr., MD, "Long-term L-Arginine Supplementation Improves Small-Vessel Coronary Endothelial Function in Humans," *Circulation* 97 (1998): 2123-28.

Jared M. Dickinson, Christopher S. Fry, Micah J. Drummond, David M. Gundermann, Dillon K. Walker, Erin L. Glynn, Kyle L. Timmerman, Shaheen Dhanani, Elena Volpi, and Blake B. Rasmussen, "Mammalian Target of Rapamycin Complex 1 Activation Is Required for the Stimulation of Human Skeletal Muscle Protein Synthesis by Essential Amino Acids," *The Journal of Nutrition* 141, no. 5 (1 May 2011): 856-62.

Chapter 6

Mayo Clinic staff, "Strength training: Get stronger, leaner, healthier," http://www.mayoclinic.com.

Judy E. Anderson, "A Role for Nitric Oxide in Muscle Repair: Nitric Oxide-mediated Activation of Muscle Satellite Cells," *Molecular Biology of the Cell* 11 (May 2000): 1859-74.

M. Matejovic, P. Radermacher, I. Tugtekin, et al., "Effects of selective iNOS inhibition on gut and liver O2-exchange and energy metabolism during hyperdynamic porcine endotoxemia," *Shock* 16, no. 3 (2001): 203-10.

M.A. Tarnopolsky, J.D. MacDougall, and S.A. Atkinson, "Influence of protein intake and training status on nitrogen balance and lean body mass," *Journal of Applied Physiology* 64, no. 1 (January 1988): 187-93.

M.L. Fernandez, "Dietary cholesterol provided by eggs and plasma lipoproteins in healthy populations," *Current Opinion in Clinical Nutrition & Metabolic Care* 9 (2006): 8-12.

Linda Houtkooper, "Weight Gain Tips for Athletes," University of Arizona Cooperative Extension, http://cals.arizona.edu/pubs/health/az1385.pdf.

Chiung-I Chang, James C. Liao, and Lih Kuo, "Arginase modulates nitric oxide production in activated macrophages," *Heart and Circulatory Physiology* 274, no. 1 (January 1998).

Ewa Jówko, MS; Piotr Ostaszewski, DVM, PhD; Michal Jank, DVM; Jaroslaw Sacharuk, PhD; Agnieszka Zieniewicz, MS; Jacek Wilczak, PhD; and Steve Nissen, DVM, "Creatine and β-hydroxy-β-methylbutyrate (HMB) additively increase lean body mass and muscle strength during a weight-training program," *Nutrition* 17, no. 7 (July 2001): 558-66.

Jeff S. Volek, PhD, RD, and Eric S. Rawson, PhD, "Scientific basis and practical aspects of creatine supplementation for athletes," *Nutrition* 20, no. 7 (July 2004): 609-14.

"Proteins are the Body's Worker Molecules," *The Structures of Life*, National Institute of General Medical Sciences, http://publications.nigms.nih.gov.

Jim Stoppani, Timothy Scheett, James Pena, Chuck Rudolph, and Derek Charlebois, "Consuming a supplement containing branched-chain amino acids during a resistance-training program increases lean mass, muscle strength and fat loss," *Journal of the International Society of Sports Nutrition* 6, no. 1 (2009): 1.

E. Roth et al., "Metabolic Disorders in Severe Abdominal Sepsis, Glutamine Deficiency in Skeletal Muscle," *Clinical Nutrition* 1 (1982): 25-41.

Joe Klemczewski, "Glutamine," (2002): http://www.joesrevolution.com.

Chapter 7

Louis Ignarro, PhD, "To Your Heart Health," http://www.edietstar.com.

F.J. Larsen, E. Weitzberg, J.O. Lundberg, and B. Ekblom, "Effects of dietary nitrate on oxygen cost during exercise," *Acta Physiologica* 191, no. 1 (September 2007) 59–66.

M.W. Radomski, R.M.J. Palmer, and S. Moncada, "Endogenous Nitric Oxide Inhibits Human Platelet Adhesion To Vascular Endothelium," *The Lancet* 330, no. 8567 (7 November 1987): 1057-58.

M. Silvia Taga, E.E. Miller and D.E. Pratt, "Chia seeds as a source of natural lipid antioxidants," *Journal of the American Oil Chemists Society* 61, no. 5: 928-31.

S.J. Bailey, P. Winyard, A. Vanhatalo, J.R. Blackwell, F.J. Dimenna, D.P. Wilkerson, J. Tarr, and N. Benjamin, A.M. Jones, "Dietary nitrate supplementation reduces the O2 cost of low-intensity exercise and enhances tolerance to high-intensity exercise in humans," *Journal of Applied Physiology* 107, no. 4 (October 2009): 1144-55.

S.J. Bailey et al., "Influence of N-acetylcysteine administration on pulmonary O2 uptake kinetics and exercise tolerance in humans," *Respiratory Physiology & Neurobiology* 175, no. 1 (31 January 2011): 121-29.

Andrew J. Maxwell, Hoai-Ky V. Ho, Christine Q. Le, Patrick S. Lin, Daniel Bernstein, and John P. Cooke, "L-Arginine enhances aerobic exercise capacity in association with augmented nitric oxide production," *Journal of Applied Physiology* 90, no. 3 (March 2001): 933-938.

Stephen J. Bailey, Paul G. Winyard, Anni Vanhatalo, Jamie R. Blackwell, Fred J. DiMenna, Daryl P. Wilkerson, and Andrew M. Jones, "Acute L-arginine supplementation reduces the O2 cost of moderate-intensity exercise and enhances high-intensity exercise tolerance," *Journal of Applied Physiology* 109, no. 5 (November 2010): 1394-1403.

"Anti-Inflammatory Effects Of Omega 3 Fatty Acid In Fish Oil Linked To Lowering Of Prostaglandin," *Science Daily* (4 April 2006).

E. Blomstrand, P. Hassmén, S. Ek, B. Ekblom, and E.A. Newsholme, "Influence of ingesting a solution of branched-chain amino acids on perceived exertion during exercise," *Acta Physiologica Scandinavica* 159, no. 1 (January 1997): 41–49.

Darin J. Falk, Kate A. Heelan, John P. Thyfault, and Alex J. Koch, "Effects of Effervescent Creatine, Ribose, and Glutamine Supplementation on Muscular Strength, Muscular Endurance, and Body Composition," *Journal of Strength and Conditioning Research* 17, no. 4 (2003): 810–16.

Chapter 8

PsychCentral News Editor, "Sleep Deprivation Common Among Americans," reviewed by John M. Grohol, PsyD, (9 March 2010): http://www.psychcentral.com.

Mike Sweeney, "What Percentage of Body Weight Suffers When Losing Water During a Sports Performance?" http://www.livestrong.com.

Christopher S.D. Almond, MD, MPH, et al., "Hyponatremia among Runners in the Boston Marathon," *New England Journal of Medicine* 352 (2005): 1550-56.

Miguel Cavazos, "The Effects of Nitric Oxide Supplement," http://www.livestrong.com.

Santosh Shinde, PhD, et al., "Coenzyme Q10: A Review of Essential Functions," *The Internet Journal of Nutrition and Wellness* 1, no. 2 (2005).

M. Negro et al., "Branched-chain amino acid supplementation does not enhance athletic performance but affects muscle recovery and the immune system," *Journal of Sports Medicine and Physical Fitness*, 48, no. 3 (2008): 347-51.

Olu Odebunmi, "Difference Between Whey & Whey Isolate," http://www.livestrong.com.

"Post Workout Recovery," http://www.civilianmilitarycombine.com.

W.J. Kraemer, J.S. Volek, D.N. French, M.R. Rubin, M.J. Sharman, A.L. Gomez, N.A. Ratamess, R.U. Newton, B. Jemiolo, B.W. Craig, and K. Hakkinen, "The effects of L-carnitine L-tartrate supplementation on hormonal responses to resistance exercise and recovery," *Journal of Strength and Conditioning Research* 17, no. 3 (2003): 455-62.

Chapter 9

Mustafa Atalay, MD, MPH, PhD; Jani Lappalainen, PhD; Chandan K. Sen, PhD, "Nutrition Dietary Antioxidants for the Athlete," *Current Sports Medicine Reports* 5, no. 4 (August 2006): 182-86.

A.K. Adams and T.M. Best, "The Role of Antioxidants in Exercise and Disease Prevention," *The Physician and Sportsmedicine* 30, no. 5 (May 2002): 37-46.

Susan M. Kleiner, PhD, RD, "Antioxidants: Vitamins That Do Battle," *Physician and Sportsmedicine* 22, no. 2 (February 1994): 23-24.

P.M. Clarkson and H.S. Thompson, "Antioxidants: What Role Do They Play in Physical Activity and Health?" *American Journal of Clinical Nutrition* 72, no. 2 (2000): 637S-646S.

Rex Rhein, "Antioxidants Let Weekend Athletes Avoid Soreness," *Family Practice News* (1 August 1996): 32.

Tommi J. Vasankari, "Increased serum and low-density-lipoprotein antioxidant potential after antioxidant supplementation in endurance athletes," *The American Journal of Clinical Nutrition* 65 (1997): 1052-56.

A.S. Rousseau and I. Margaritis, "Physical activity alters antioxidant status in exercising elderly subjects," *The Journal of Nutritional Biochemistry* 17, no. 7 (2006): 463-70.

J. Louis, C. Hausswirth, F. Bieuzen, and J. Brisswalter, "Vitamin and mineral supplementation effect on muscular activity and cycling efficiency in master athletes," *Applied Physiology, Nutrition, and Metabolism* 35, no. 3 (June 2010): 251-60.

O. Neubauer, S. Reichhold, L. Nics, C. Hoelzl, J. Valentini, B. Stadlmayr, S. Knasmüller, and K.H. Wagner, "Antioxidant responses to an acute ultra-endurance exercise: impact on DNA stability and indications for an increased need for nutritive antioxidants in the early recovery phase," *British Journal of Nutrition* 104, no. 8 (Oct. 2010): 1129-38.

E.M. Peters, J.M. Goetzsche, and B. Grobbelaar, "Vitamin C supplementation reduces the incidence of postrace symptoms of upper-respiratory-tract infection in ultramarathon runners," *American Journal of Clinical Nutrition* 57 (1993): 170-74.

P. Tauler, A. Aguiló, E. Fuentespina, J. Tur, and A. Pons, "Diet supplementation with vitamin E, vitamin C and ß-carotene cocktail enhances basal neutrophil antioxidant enzymes in athletes," *European Journal of Physiology* 443, no. 5-6 (2002): 791-97.

Jean-Claude Guilland, Thierry Penaranda, Corinne Gallet, Vincent Boggio, Françoise Fuchs, and Jacques Klepping, "Vitamin status of young athletes including the effects of supplementation," *Medicine & Science in Sports & Exercise* (2007).

C.J. Krumbach, D.R. Ellis, and J.A. Driskell, "A report of vitamin and mineral supplement use among University athletes in a Division I Institution," *International Journal of Sport Nutrition* 9, no. 4 (1999): 416-25.

Jonathan M. Peake, "Vitamin C: Effects of Exercise and Requirements With Training," *International Journal of Sport Nutrition and Exercise Metabolism* 13 (2003): 125-51.

H. Gerster, "The role of Vitamin C in athletic performance," *American College of Nutrition* 8, no. 6 (December 1989): 636-43.

William J. Evans, "Vitamin E, vitamin C, and exercise 1, 2, 3," *American Journal of Clinical Nutrition* 72, no. 2 (August 2000): 647S-652S.

S. Patlar and E. Boyali, "Elements in Sera of Elite Taekwondo Athletes: Effects of Vitamin E Supplementation," *Biological Trace Element Research* 139, no. 2 (February 2011): 119-25.

P.M. Tiidus and M.E. Houston, "Vitamin E status and response to exercise training," *Sports Medicine* 20, no. 1 (July 1995): 12-23.

Y. Hellsten and J.J. Nielsen, "Antioxidant supplementation enhances the exercise-induced increase in mitochondrial uncoupling protein 3 and endothelial nitric oxide synthase mRNA content in human skeletal muscle," *Free Radical Biology and Medicine* 43, no. 3 (2007): 353-61.

Jennifer M. Sacheck, Eric A. Decker, and Priscilla M. Clarkson, "The effect of diet on Vitamin E intake and oxidative stress in response to acute exercise in female athletes," *European Journal of Applied Physiology* 83, no. 1 (September 2000): 40-46.

R.J. Shephard, R. Campbell, P. Pimm, D. Stuart, and G.R. Wright, "Vitamin E, exercise, and the recovery from physical activity," *European Journal of Applied Physiology and Occupational Physiology* 33, no. 2: 119-26.

G. Haralambie, "Serum Zinc in Athletes in Training," *International Journal of Sports Medicine* 2, no. 3 (1981): 135-38.

MScM. Fogelholm, MScJ. Laakso, MScJ. Lehto, and BAI. Ruokonen, "Dietary intake and indicators of magnesium and zinc status in male athletes," *Nutrition Research* 11, no. 10 (October 1991): 1111-18.

L.M. Weight, T.D. Noakes, D. Labadarios, J. Graves, P. Jacobs, and P.A. Berman, "Vitamin and mineral status of trained athletes including the effects of supplementation," *American Journal of Clinical Nutrition* 47, no. 2 (February 1988): 186-91.

T.D. Fahey, J.D. Larsen, G.A. Brooks, W. Colvin, S. Henderson, and D. Lary, "The effects of ingesting polylactate or glucose polymer drinks during prolonged exercise," *International Journal of Sport Nutrition* 1, no. 3 (September 1991): 249-56.

George Brooks, "What Is Polylactate And What Does It Do?" Mass Nutrition, http://www.mass.fi/article.asp?id=68.

John L. Azevedo, Jr., Emily Tietz, Tashena Two-Feathers, Jeff Paull, and Kenneth Chapman, "Lactate, Fructose and Glucose Oxidation Profiles in Sports Drinks and the Effect on Exercise Performance," *PLoS One* 2, no. 9 (26 September 2007): e927.
Thomas D. Fahey, James D. Larsen, George A. Brooks, Steven Henderson, and Darrel Lary, "The Effects of Ingesting Polylactate or Glucose Polymer Drinks During Prolonged Exercise," *Sports and Nutrition* 1, no. 3 (September 1991): 249-56.

Chapter 10

Håkan K. R. Karlsson, Per-Anders Nilsson, Johnny Nilsson, Alexander V. Chibalin, Juleen R. Zierath, and Eva Blomstrand, "Branched-chain amino acids increase p70S6k phosphorylation in human skeletal muscle after resistance exercise," *American Journal of Physiology – Endocrinology and Metabolism* 287, no. 1 (July 2004): E1-E7.

Jason E. Tang, Daniel R. Moore, Gregory W. Kujbida, Mark A. Tarnopolsky, and Stuart M. Phillip, "Ingestion of whey hydrolysate, casein, or soy protein isolate: effects on mixed muscle protein synthesis at rest and following resistance exercise in young men," *Physiology* 107, no. 3 (September 2009): 987-92.

L.Q. Qin et al., "Higher Branched-Chain Amino Acid Intake Is Associated with a Lower Prevalence of Being Overweight or Obese in Middle-Aged East Asian and Western Adults," *Journal of Nutrition* 141, no. 2 (February 2011): 249-54.

E.F. Palo, P. Metus, R. Gatti, O. Previti, L. Bigon, and C.B. Palo, "Branched chain amino acids chronic treatment and muscular exercise performance in athletes: a study through plasma acetyl-carnitine levels," *Amino Acids* 4, no. 3: 255-66.

E.F. De Palo, R. Gatti, E. Cappellin, C. Schiraldi, C.B. De Palo, and P. Spinella, "Plasma lactate, GH and GH-binding protein levels in exercise following BCAA supplementation in athletes," *Amino Acids* 20, no. 1: 1-11.

Reinaldo A. Bassit, Letícia A. Sawada, Reury F. Bacurau, Franciso Navarro, Eivor Martins, Jr., Ronaldo V. Santos, Erico C. Caperuto, Patrícia Rogeri, and Luís F. Costa Rosa, "Branched-chain amino acid supplementation and the immune response of long-distance athletes," *Nutrition* 18, no. 5 (May 2002): 376-79.

L. Di Luigi, Laura Guidetti, Fabio Pigozzi, Carlo Baldari, Alessandro Casini, Maurizo Nordio, and Francesco Romanelli, "Acute amino acids supplementation enhances pituitary responsiveness in athletes," *Medicine & Science in Sports & Exercise* 31, no. 12 (December 1999): 1748.

Huang Jin-li and Ou Ming-hao, "The Effect of Branched-chain Amino Acid Supplementation on Gluconeogenesis of Athletes After Exhaustive Exercise," *Journal of Tianjin University of Sport* (2006).

Chapter 11

J.M. Davis and C.J. Carlstedt, "The dietary flavonoid quercetin increases VO(2max) and endurance capacity," *International Journal of Sport Nutrition and Exercise Metabolism* 20, no. 1 (February 2010): 56-62.

H. Gökbel, I. Gül, M. Belviran, and N. Okudan, "The Effects Of Coenzyme Q10 Supplementation on Performance During Repeated Bouts of Supramaximal Exercise in Sedentary Men," *Journal of Strength and Conditioning Research* (28 July 2009).

M. Cooke and R. Kreider, "Effects of acute and 14-day coenzyme Q10 supplementation on exercise performance in both trained and untrained individuals," *Journal of the International Society of Sports Nutrition* 5, no. 1 (2008): 8.

A. Zheng and T. Moritani, "Influence of CoQ10 on Autonomic Nervous Activity and Energy Metabolism during Exercise in Healthy Subjects," *Journal of Nutritional Science and Vitaminology* (Tokyo) 54, no. 4 (2008): 286-90.

M. Konet et al., "Reducing exercise-induced muscular injury in kendo athletes with supplementation of coenzyme Q10," *British Journal of Nutrition* 100, no. 4 (2008): 903-9.

J. Islam, B.F. Uretsky, and V.S. Sierpina, "Heart failure improvement with CoQ10, Hawthorn, and magnesium in a patient scheduled for cardiac resynchronization-defibrillator therapy: a case study," *Explore* (NY) 2, no. 4 (2006): 339-41.

S. Sander and S.I. Coleman, "The impact of coenzyme Q10 on systolic function in patients with chronic heart failure," *Journal of Cardiac Failure* 12, no. 6 (2006): 464-72.

S.A. Shah and S. Sander, "Electrocardiographic and hemodynamic effects of coenzyme Q10 in healthy individuals: a double-blind, randomized controlled trial," *The Annals of Pharmacotherapy* 41, no. 3 (2007): 420-25.

Chapter 12

Paul L. Greenhaff, "Creatine and Its Applications as an Ergogenic Aid," *International Journal of Sports Nutrition* 5 (1995): S100-10.

Ronald J. Maughan, "Creatine Supplementation and Exercise Performance," *International Journal of Sports Nutrition* 5 (1995): 94-101.

Melvin H. Williams, PhD, and J. David Branch, PhD, "Creatine Supplementation and Exercise Performance: An Update," *Journal of the American College of Nutrition* 17, no. 3 (1998): 216-34.

M.W. Rich, "Chronic Heart Failure," *Handbook of Clinical Nutrition* and Aging, 437-53

Stephen M. Cornish, Darren G. Candow, Nathan T. Jantz, Philip D. Chilibeck, Jonathan P. Little, Scott Forbes, Saman Abeysekara, and Gordon A. Zello, "Conjugated Linoleic Acid Combined With Creatine Monohydrate and Whey Protein Supplementation During Strength Training," *IJSNEM* 19, no. 1 (February 2009).

Jonathan P. Little, Scott C. Forbes, Darren G. Candow, Stephen M. Cornish, and Philip D. Chilibeck, "Creatine, Arginine α-Ketoglutarate, Amino Acids, and Medium-Chain Triglycerides and Endurance and Performance," *IJSNEM* 18, no. 5 (October 2008).

R.B. Kreider, "Creatine, the Next Ergogenic Supplement?" *Sportscience Training & Technology*, Internet Society for Sport Science (2008).

Konstantinos Havenetidis, Ourania Matsouka, Carlton Brian Cooke, and Apostolos Theodorou, "The use of varying creatine regimens on sprintcycling," *Journal of Sports Science and Medicine* 2 (2003): 88-97.

M.A. Tarnopolsky and D.P. MacLennan, "Creatine monohydrate supplementation enhances high-intensity exercise performance in males and females," *International Journal of Sport Nutrition and Exercise Metabolism* 10, no. 4 (2000): 452-63.

M.D. Becque, J.D. Lochmann, and D.R. Melrose, "Effects of oral creatine supplementation on muscular strength and body composition," *Medicine & Science in Sports & Exercise* 32, no. 3 (2000): 654-58..

John M. Lawler, William S. Barnes, Gaoyao Wu, Wook Song, and Scott Demaree, "Direct Antioxidant Properties of Creatine," *Biochemical and Biophysical Research Communications* 290 (2002): 47–52.

K.L. Kendall, A.E. Smith, J.L. Graef, D.H. Fukuda, J.R. Moon, T.W. Beck, J.T. Cramer, and J.R. Stout, "Effects of four weeks of high-intensity interval training and creatine supplementation on critical power and anaerobic working capacity in college-aged men," *Journal of Strength & Conditioning Research* 23, no. 6 (September 2009): 1663-69.

J.Y. Ho, W.J. Kraemer, J.S. Volek, M.S. Fragala, G.A. Thomas, C. Dunn-Lewis, M. Coday, K. Häkkinen, and C.M. Maresh, "L-Carnitine l-tartrate supplementation favorably affects biochemical markers of recovery from physical exertion in middle-aged men and women," *Metabolism* (30 December 2009).

J.L. Graef, A.E. Smith, K.L. Kendall, D.H. Fukuda, J.R. Moon, T.W. Beck, J.T. Cramer, and J.R. Stout, "The effects of four weeks of creatine supplementation and high-intensity interval training on cardiorespiratory fitness: a randomized controlled trial," *Journal of the International Society of Sports Nutrition* 6 (2009): 18

Y.L. Law, W.S. Ong, T.L. GillianYap, S.C. Lim, and E. Von Chia, "Effects of two and five days of creatine loading on muscular strength and anaerobic power in trained athletes," *Journal of Strength & Conditioning Research* 23, no. 3 (May 2009): 906-14.

A.P. Johnston, D.G. Burke, L.G. MacNeil, and D.G. Candow, "Effect of creatine supplementation during cast-induced immobilization on the preservation of muscle mass, strength, and endurance," *Journal of Strength & Conditioning Research* 23, no. 1 (January 2009): 116-20.

Chapter 13

U.N. Das, "Essential Fatty Acids and Osteoporosis," *Nutrition* 16 (2000): 386-90. .

B. Tartibian and B.H. Maleki, "Omega-3 Fatty acids supplementation attenuates inflammatory markers after eccentric exercise in untrained men," *Clinical Journal of Sport Medicine* 21, no. 2 (March 2011): 131-37.

Timothy D. Mickleborough, Rachael L. Murray, Alina A. Ionescu, and Martin R. Lindley, "Fish Oil Supplementation Reduces Severity of Exercise-Induced Bronchoconstriction in Elite Athletes," *American Journal of Respiratory and Critical Care Medicine* 168 (2003): 1181-89.

R. Carmena, MD, and S.M. Grundy, MD, "Management of Hypertriglyceridemic Patients. B. Dietary Management of Hypertriglyceridemic Patients," *The American Journal of Cardiology* 68 (24 July 1991): 35A-37A.

D. König, A. Berg, C. Weinstock, J. Keul, and H. Northoff, "Essential fatty acids, immune function, and exercise," *Exercise Immunology* Review 3 (1997): 1-31.

Chapter 14

C.L. Camic, T.J. Housh, J.M. Zuniga, R.C. Hendrix, M. Mielke, G.O. Johnson, and R.J. Schmidt, "Effects of Arginine-Based Supplements on the Physical Working Capacity at the Fatigue Threshold," *The Journal of Strength & Conditioning Research* 24, no. 5 (May 2010): 1306-12.

Jonathan P. Little, Scott C. Forbes, Darren G. Candow, Stephen M. Cornish, and Philip D. Chilibeck, "Creatine, Arginine α-Ketoglutarae, Amino Acids, and Medium-Chain Triglycerides and Endurance and Performance," *IJSNEM* 18, no. 5 (October 2008).

Ben B. Yaspelkis III and John L. Ivy, "The Effect of a Carbohydrate—Arginine Supplement on Postexercise Carbohydrate Metabolism," *IJSNEM* 20, no. 4 (November 2009).

A. Schaefer and F. Piquard, "L-Arginine Reduces Exercise-Induced Increase in Plasma Lactate and Ammonia," *International Journal of Sports Medicine* 23 (2002): 403-7.

Leszek Ceremuzynski, MD, PhD, "Effect of Supplemental Oral L-Arginine on Exercise Capacity in Patients With Stable Angina Pectoris," *The American Journal of Cardiology* 80 (1 August 1997): 331-33.

N. Nagaya, M. Uematsu, and H. Oya, "Short-Term Oral Administration of L-Arginine Improves Hemodynamics and Exercise Capacity in Patients With Precapillary Pulmonary Hypertension," *American Journal of Respiratory and Critical Care Medicine* 163 (2001): 887-91.

Chapter 15

A. Figueroa and F. Vicil, "Oral L-Citrulline Supplementation Attenuates Blood Pressure Response to Cold Pressor Test in Young Men," *American Journal of Hypertension* (22 October 2009).
K. Sasajima, "Increases in pulmonary artery pressure and cardiac output due to the inhibition of nitric oxide synthesis during operative stress," *Journal Surgery Today* 25, no. 10 (October 2005).

Arturo Figueroa, Julian A. Trivino, Marcos A. Sanchez-Gonzalez, and Vicil Florence, "Oral L-Citrulline Supplementation Attenuates Blood Pressure Response to Cold Pressor Test in Young Men," *American Journal of Hypertension* 23, no. 1 (2010): 12–16.

Antoni Sureda, Alfredo Córdova, Miguel D. Ferrer, Pedro Tauler, Gerardo Pérez, Josep A. Tur, and Antoni Pon, "Effects of L-citrulline oral supplementation on polymorphonuclear neutrophils oxidative burst and nitric oxide production after exercise," *Informa Health Care* 43, no. 9 (2009): 828-35.

William J. Kraemer, Disa L. Hatfield, Barry A. Spiering, Jakob L. Vingren, Maren S. Fragala, Jen-Yu Ho, Jeff S. Volek, Jeffrey M. Anderson, and Carl M. Maresh, "Effects of a multi-nutrient supplement on exercise performance and hormonal responses to resistance exercise," *European Journal of Applied Physiology* 101, no. 5 (November 2007): 637-646.

M.D. Brown, M. Srinivasan, R.V. Hogikyan, D.R. Dengel1, S.G. Glickman, A. Galecki, and M.A. Supiano, "Nitric Oxide Biomarkers Increase During Exercise-Induced Vasodilation in the Forearm," *International Journal of Sports Medicine* 21, no. 2 (2000): 83-89.

Chapter 16

John T. Brosnan, "Interorgan Amino Acid Transport and its Regulation," *The Journal of Nutrition* 133 (June 2003): 2068S-72S.

P. Newsholme, M.M. Lima, J. Procopio, T.C. Pithon-Curi, S.Q. Doi, R.B. Bazotte and R. Curi, "Glutamine and glutamate as vital metabolites," *Brazilian Journal of Medical and Biological Research* 36, no. 2 (February 2003): 153-63.

Philip Newsholme, "Why Is L-Glutamine Metabolism Important to Cells of the Immune System in Health, Postinjury, Surgery or Infection?" *The Journal of Nutrition* 131, no. 9 (1 September 2001): 2515S-22S.

Wha-Joon Lee, Richard A. Hawkins, Juan R. Viña, and Darryl R. Peterson, "Glutamine transport by the blood-brain barrier a possible mechanism for nitrogen removal," *American Journal of Physiology – Cell Physiology* 274, no. 4 (April 1998): C1101-7.

Timothy C. Ballard, MD; Ahmed Farag, MD; Gene D. Branum, MD; Onye E. Akwari, MD; and Emmanuel C. Opara, PhD, "Effect of L-glutamine supplementation on impaired glucose regulation during intravenous lipid administration," *The International Journal of Applied and Basic Nutritional Sciences* 12, no. 5 (May 1996): 349-54.

Robert J. Smith, MD, "Glutamine Metabolism and Its Physiologic Importance," *Journal of Parenteral and Enteral Nutrition* 14, no. 4 (July 1990): 40S-44S.
Linda M. Castell and Eric A. Newsholme, "The effects of oral glutamine supplementation on athletes after prolonged, exhaustive exercise," *Nutrition* 13, no. 7-8 (July-August 1997): 738-42.

L.M. Castell, J.R. Poortmans, R. Leclercq, M. Brasseur, J. Duchateau, and E.A. Newsholme, "Some aspects of the acute phase response after a marathon race, and the effects of glutamine supplementation," *European Journal of Applied Physiology and Occupational Physiology* 75, no. 1 (1997): 47-53.

Jose Antonio and Chris Street, "Glutamine: A Potentially Useful Supplement for Athletes," *Canadian Journal of Applied Physiology* 24, no. 1 (1999): 1-14.

Chapter 17

Rosa Huertas, Yolanda Campos, Enrique Díaz, Jesus Esteban, Leonardo Vechietti, Giussepe Montanari, Stefania D'Iddio, Marco Corsi, and Joaquin Arenas, "Respiratory chain enzymes in muscle of endurance athletes: Effect of L-carnitine," *Biochemical and Biophysical Research Communications* 188, no. 1 (15 October 1992): 102-7.

C. Marconi, G. Sassi, A. Carpinelli, and P. Cerretelli, "Effects of L-carnitine loading on the aerobic and anaerobic performance of endurance athletes," *European Journal of Applied Physiology and Occupational Physiology* 54, no. 2 (1985): 131-35.

R. Nüesch, M. Rosstto, and B. Martina, "Plasma and urine carnitine concentrations in well-trained athletes at rest and after exercise, Influence of L-carnitine intake," *Drugs Under Experimental & Clinical Research* 25, no. 4 (1999): 167-71.

C.P. Cerretelli, "L-Carnitine Supplementation in Humans, The Effects on Physical Performance," *International Journal of Sports Medicine* 11, no. 1 (1990): 1-14.

Paolo Colombani, Caspar Wenk, Iris Kunz, Stephan Krähenbühl, Martina Kuhnt, Myrtha Arnold, Petra Frey-Rindova, Walter Frey, and Wolfgang Langhans, "Effects of L-carnitine supplementation on physical performance and energy metabolism of endurance-trained athletes: a double-blind crossover field study," *European Journal of Applied Physiology and Occupational Physiology* 73, no. 5 (1996): 434-39

Heidrun Karlic, PhD, and Alfred Lohninger, PhD, "Supplementation of L-carnitine in athletes," *Nutrition* 20, no. 7-8 (July-August 2004): 709-15.

Eric P. Brass, "Supplemental carnitine and exercise," *American Journal of Clinical Nutrition* (August 2000) 72, no. 2: 618S-23S.

K.H. Schulpis, T. Parthimos, E.D. Papakonstantinou, T. Tsakiris, N. Parthimos, A.F. Mentis, and S. Tsakiris, "Evidence for the participation of the stimulated sympathetic nervous system in the regulation of carnitine blood levels of soccer players during a game," *Metabolism* 58, no. 8 (August 2009): 1080-86.

M. Gacek, "Eating habits of a group of professional volleyball players," *Rocz Panstw Zakl Hig* 62, no. 1 (2011): 77-82.

A. Berg, "Vitamin supplements, protein preparations, carnitine and Co. What is the benefit for amateur athletes (interview by Dr. Ulrich Scharmer)," *MMW - Fortschritte der Medizin* 144, no. 17 (25 April 2002): 14.

Chapter 18

L. Holm and J.L. Olesen, "Protein-containing nutrient supplementation following strength training enhances the effect on muscle mass, strength, and bone formation in postmenopausal women," *Journal of Applied Physiology* 105, no. 1 (2008): 274-81.

R.B. Kreider, V. Miriel, and E. Bertun, "Amino Acid Supplementation and Exercise Performance: Analysis of the Proposed Ergogenic Value," *Sports Medicine* 16, no. 3 (1993): 190-209.

I. Elmadfa and B. Rupp, "Nutritional Status of Young Athletes," *Bibliotheca Nutritio et Dieta* 51 (1994): 163-65.

Elizabeth Quinn, "Sports Nutrition - Protein Needs for Athletes," *About.com Sports Medicine* (2 December 2007): http://sportsmedicine.about.com/od/sportsnutrition/a/Protein.htm.

Bill Campbell, Richard B. Kreider, Tim Ziegenfuss, Paul La Bounty, Mike Roberts, Darren Burke, Jamie Landis, Hector Lopez, and Jose Antonio, "International Society of Sports Nutrition position stand: protein and exercise," *Journal of the International Society of Sports Nutrition* 4 (2007): 8.

L.J.C. van Loon, A.K. Kies, and W.H.M. Saris, "Protein and Protein Hydrolysates in Sports Nutrition," *IJSNEM* 17 (August 2007): S1-S4.

Melissa J. Benton and Pamela D. Swan, "Effect of Protein Ingestion on Energy Expenditure and Substrate Utilization After Exercise in Middle-Aged Women," *IJSNEM* 17, no. 6 (December 2007).

Paul J. Arciero, Christopher L. Gentile, Roger Martin-Pressman, Michael J. Ormsbee, Meghan Everett, Lauren Zwicky, and Christine A. Steele, "Increased Dietary Protein and Combined High Intensity Aerobic and Resistance Exercise Improves Body Fat Distribution and Cardiovascular Risk Factors," *IJSNEM* 16, no. 4 (August 2006).

John G. Seifert, Joseph Harmon, and Patty DeClercq, "Protein Added to a Sports Drink Improves Fluid Retention," *IJSNEM* 16, no. 4 (August 2006).

Ryan D. Andrews, David A. MacLean, and Steven E. Riechman, "Protein Intake for Skeletal Muscle Hypertrophy with Resistance Training in Seniors," *IJSNEM* 16, no. 2 (April 2006).

Paolo C. Colombani, Eva M. R. Kovacs, Petra Frey-Rindova, Walter Frey, Wolfgang Langhans, Myrtha Arnold, and Caspar Wenk, "Metabolic Effects of a Protein-Supplemented Carbohydrate Drink in Marathon Runners," *IJSNEM* 9, no. 2 (June 1999).

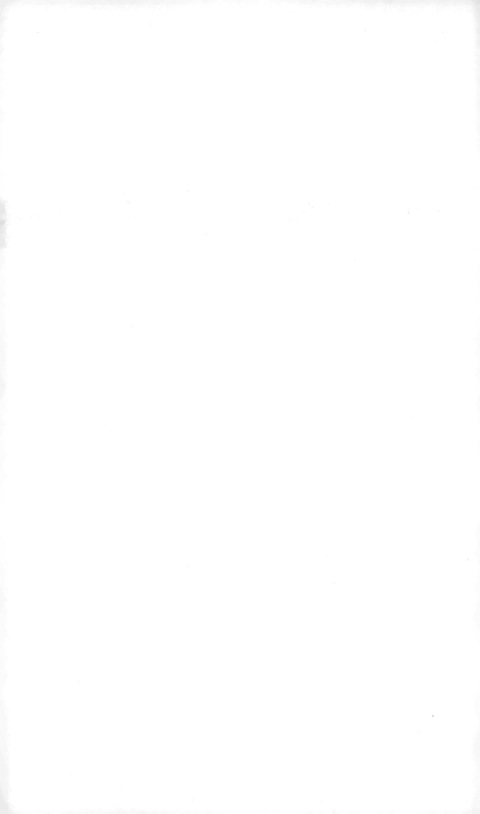

Acknowledgements

It takes many supportive people to give life to a concept and book like *Health is Wealth.* To each and every person that has been a part of the development of this book; we would like to offer a humble and heartfelt, "Thank you!"

Thank you as well, to the readers of this book who believe that "*healthcare is really self-care*" and are willing to help share our wellness message with their families, friends, and coworkers. We wrote *Health is Wealth* for the purpose of empowering our readers to take charge of their own wellness and make a positive and lasting impact on their quality of life.

Our deepest thanks to:

Our families and friends for their constant love and support throughout the book development process.

Our friend and business partner, Dave Brubaker, whose entrepreneurial spirit and business acumen helps to guide our success.

Our *Health is Wealth* book production and online team: Denny Hooten for his professionalism, humor, and the expansion of the *Health is Wealth* concept and brand. Landon Wackerli for jumping in and making things happen; Maryanna Young for her friendship, leadership, and project management; Shannon Tracy for her research, support, and keeping up with the health science side of this project; Amy Meyer for her constant support and dedicated hard work; Hillary Hunnewell for her commitment to great products and for the massive amount of effort she puts into everything she does. Thanks to Cari Campbell for cover design; Tim Vandehey for interviewing and writing skills; Nick and Betsy Zelinger at NZ Graphics for interior design and editing; Lloyd Jassin for legal advice and direction; Stacy Ennis, Amy Breuggemann, Morgan Barry, and Kathy McIntosh for proofreading and final polishing of our content. Thanks to Patty Murphy and Sandra Rea for their help in the early stages of Performance Nutrition. Stephen Watts and Kelly Antonczak, thanks for continuing to bring messages to the online *Health is Wealth* community.

SPREAD THE WEALTH!

Health is Wealth books are available at quantity discounts for orders of 10 or more copies. Additional volume discounts apply for quantities of 100, 500 or 1000.

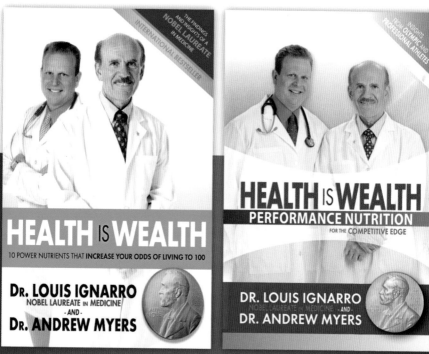

ISBN 978-0-9790229-1-3

ISBN 978-1-61-389-002-8

To find out about our discounts on orders of 10 or more copies for individuals, corporations, academic use, associations and organizations, please call us at (800) 817-0018 or visit our web site, healthiswealth.net.

To find out about our discount program for resellers, please contact our Special Sales department at lwackerli@nutragenetics.net.

From the Authors of
HEALTH IS WEALTH

TWO OTHER GREAT EDUCATIONAL CHOICES
WITH REGARDS TO IMPROVING YOUR HEALTH AND WELLNESS!

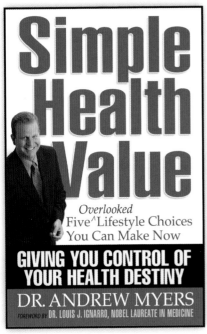

ISBN 978-0-9790229-1-6

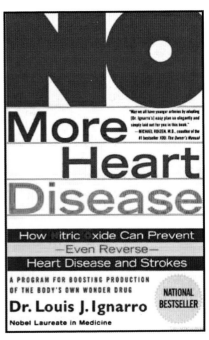

ISBN 0-312-3358-2-2

On **NO More Heart Disease,** Michael Roizen, MD,
coauthor of the #1 bestseller *YOU: The Owner's Manual,* offers:

**"May we all have younger arteries by adopting Dr. Ignarro's
easy plan so elegantly and simply laid out in this book."**

On *Simple Health Value*, Bill Sears, MD, America's Pediatrician, offers:
**"A highly-recommended must-read.
Regardless of what you're doing to improve your health,
this book will help you to feel and look your best."**

To find out about our discounts for orders of 10 or more copies for
individuals, corporations, academic use, associations and organizations,
please call us at (800) 817-0018 or visit our web site, healthiswealth.net.

To find out about our discount program for resellers, please contact our
Special Sales department at lwackerli@nutragenetics.net.

HEALTH IS WEALTH.NET

- Learn how to enter our **monthly giveaways.**
- Subscribe to the **Health Is Wealth newsletter.**
- Visit the **Doctors' Orders Blog** to learn more about a healthy lifestyle.
- Purchase books and **watch free videos.**
- Read what we've heard from others like you.
- Send us your comments and thoughts on Health is Wealth.
- Follow us on **facebook** and **twitter.**

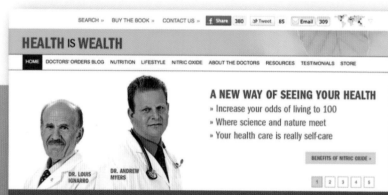

SEARCH »   BUY THE BOOK »   CONTACT US »   Share 380   Tweet 85   Email 309

HEALTH IS WEALTH

HOME | DOCTORS' ORDERS BLOG | NUTRITION | LIFESTYLE | NITRIC OXIDE | ABOUT THE DOCTORS | RESOURCES | TESTIMONIALS | STORE

A NEW WAY OF SEEING YOUR HEALTH
» Increase your odds of living to 100
» Where science and nature meet
» Your health care is really self-care

BENEFITS OF NITRIC OXIDE »

1 2 3 4 5

DR. LOUIS IGNARRO   DR. ANDREW MYERS

HEALTH IS WEALTH: LEARN TO LIVE LONGER

Nobel Laureate in Medicine Dr. Louis Ignarro and Naturopathic Physician Dr. Andrew Myers have teamed up to transform forever how you think about disease and health. Our goal is to save lives and prevent illness through science and nutrition. By changing your perspective, you will change your choices, and better choices will lead to a thrilling enhancement of your wellness, energy, and longevity. What if you could avoid disease simply by promoting the optimal function of your body? What if we redefined disease? What if disease was not the inevitable end-point of our lives, but that, if properly supported, the body would continue to function optimally even at an advanced age? Explore our site to find out more. To quote Ralph Waldo Emerson: The first wealth is health.

Buy the book and learn how to live to 100!

ORDER NOW »

SIGN UP FREE: HEALTH ALERTS

Our Health Is Wealth: Health Alerts will help you live to 100! Receive our free informational email alerts with health tips and learn how to enter our monthly giveaways. You too can read what *we* are reading, every week!

Sign up now, its free! »

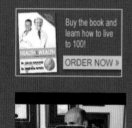

0:00 / 0:00
WATCH MORE V

DOCTORS' ORDER

Scan with smart phone